BIT7

BITTER SEA
The Human Cost of
Minamata Disease

by
Akio Mishima

translated by
Richard L. Gage
and
Susan B. Murata

with a foreword by
Lester R. Brown

KOSEI PUBLISHING CO. • *Tokyo*

This book was originally published in Japanese under the title *Nake, Shiranui no Umi: Minamata ni Sasageta Chinkon no Tatakai*, © 1977 by Akio Mishima.

The cover photograph shows Jitsuko Tanaka, thirty-three years old when this photograph was taken in 1986. Born to a family of shipwrights, she contracted Minamata disease in 1956, at the age of three. Four members of her family have fallen victim to the disease, including both her parents. Jitsuko cannot talk, and she can walk only with assistance. Her hands exhibit the deformity typical of Minamata disease. Her oldest sister helps her totter along the wharf near her home on Minamata Bay. Jitsuko wears the brightly colored, long-sleeved kimono of a young unmarried woman, which she will always be, whatever her chronological age. This photograph is by Shisei Kuwabara.

Editing by EDS Inc., Editorial & Design Services, Tokyo. Book design, typography, layout of photographs, and cover design by Becky Davis, EDS Inc. The text of this book is set in Monotype Baskerville, with Monotype Baskerville for display.

First English edition, 1992

Published by Kosei Publishing Co., Kosei Building, 2-7-1 Wada, Suginami-ku, Tokyo 166, Japan. Copyright © 1992 by Kosei Publishing Co.; all rights reserved. Printed in Japan.

ISBN 4-333-01479-4   LCC Card No. applied for

CONTENTS

Map faces page 18
Photographs follow page 72

FOREWORD

Akio Mishima deserves a great deal of credit for writing *Bitter Sea: The Human Cost of Minamata Disease.* And Richard L. Gage and Susan B. Murata have done an exceptional job of translating it into English, thus bringing it to a far wider readership.

Bitter Sea is an in-depth case study painfully chronicling the struggle between the victims of Minamata disease (mercury poisoning) and the corporation that discharged the mercury into Minamata Bay. It is a gripping account of how the victims and their friends and sympathizers organized to seek justice. It is discouraging to see that the government is sometimes less interested in protecting the victims than those who are responsible for their plight.

One's heart goes out to the victims of this disabling, disfiguring disease. From *Bitter Sea,* one gets a clear idea of the scale of the disease: more than 900 deaths from Minamata disease to date; more than 2,000 patients certified; another 3,000 awaiting certification so they can collect benefits.

At times, in reading this book, one has the feeling of reading a novel, so dramatic is the account. Unfortunately, it is not fiction. It is a real-life story of how callous corporate greed can cause enormous human suffering.

This chronicle will give hope to others who are involved in similar, often protracted, conflicts.

A quick survey shows numerous examples of how the behavior of corporations or, in the case of centrally planned economies, government agencies can harm the very people they are supposed to serve. Official figures from Moscow, for example, indicate that 300,000 Russians are now being treated for radiation, and only some are victims of Chernobyl.

Johns Manville, a U.S.-based manufacturer of asbestos products, has settled some 13,000 lawsuits as a result of lung cancer and other health effects of exposure to asbestos, at a cost of $15 million. It still faces some 93,000 additional claims. Unable to satisfy all of these claims, the firm has declared bankruptcy.

Perhaps the most dramatic example of corporate disregard for human health concerns the effects of cigarette smoking. The U.S. surgeon general reports that 360,000 Americans die each year from smoking cigarettes, almost 1,000 deaths a day. Smoking now accounts for 26 percent of all cancer deaths in the United States. But more striking is the even larger number dying from heart disease and strokes as a result of smoking. Despite this officially estimated loss of almost 1,000 American lives a day, more than all the victims of Minamata disease to date, the manufacture and marketing of these highly lethal cigarettes continues. When will it stop?

One could cite a long list of instances in which irresponsible corporate behavior has led to disease and death. Akio Mishima's story of the victims of Minamata disease gives hope that socially destructive corporate behavior will be challenged on every front. To permit corporate greed to override our concern for human health is to challenge our credentials as a civilized society.

LESTER R. BROWN
President, Worldwatch Institute

Introduction to the
English Edition

The environmental threats confronting the earth today —depletion of the ozone layer, global warming due to the greenhouse effect, radioactive fallout from nuclear accidents, acid rain, destruction of rain forests, desertification, pollution of the world's waters—are of unprecedented gravity. Representatives of the family of humanity from all nations must work together to resolve these problems before it is too late, while the earth still has the power of self-restoration. To ensure the continued existence of the human race we must carry out a global environmental conservation program, converting the rule of military might to a hegemony of greenery.

Investment in the environment is certain to pay off in the long run. Sluggishness in instituting environmental policies, on the other hand, will lead to irreversible damage. A tragic example is the mercury pollution of the waters of Minamata Bay in Kumamoto Prefecture, on the west coast of the Japanese island of Kyushu.

As a result of the bay's pollution with toxic organic mercury, many people were stricken with a terrible syndrome in the 1950s. Minamata disease, as it came to be known, is characterized by numbness of the extremities and the area around the mouth, constriction of the field of vision, loss of hearing, motor and speech disorders, loss of muscle coordination, convulsions, and sometimes mental aberrations. People congenitally afflicted with the disease are often mentally retarded.

In the 1950s, when Japan was entering a phase of rapid economic growth, a manufacturer of industrial chemicals known as Chisso was the largest producer of vinyl chlorides in the nation. Its production process called for the use of large quantities of mercury as a catalyst. Goaded by the desire for ever greater production and profits, the company polluted the waters near its plant in Minamata with mercury; this was later confirmed as the cause of Minamata disease.

In the mid-1950s Dr. Hajime Hosokawa, director of the hospital attached to Chisso's Minamata plant, noticed a series of patients afflicted with a painful condition that seemed to combine the symptoms of epilepsy and paralysis. Suspecting that factory effluent might be the cause, in July 1959 he began conducting experiments in which effluent from the Minamata plant was sprinkled on food fed to cats. In October that year one of the cats was stricken with motor disorders and convulsions exactly like those exhibited by victims of the strange new illness. Examination of brain-tissue samples from the animal at Kyushu University's pathology laboratory revealed the degeneration of the cerebellum characteristic of Minamata disease.

When Hosokawa reported his findings to Chisso executives, they ordered him to halt his experiments and had the remaining cats destroyed in the utmost secrecy. Hosokawa then appealed directly to the president of the firm, Kiichi Yoshioka, for permission to continue his experiments and to publish the results, in keeping with the company's social responsibility. His request was turned down. Disillusioned, Hosokawa resigned from Chisso in 1962. In 1970, when he was terminally ill with cancer, he finally revealed what had occurred in 1959, testifying from his hospital bed in one of the trials that grew out of the Minamata problem.

Suppressing all word of the experiments though fully aware of their ominous results, Chisso continued to pump five hundred tons of poisonous effluent an hour into Minamata Bay, the source of the fish and other seafood on which the local people relied for their livelihood. Chisso refused to comply with Minamata-disease patients' requests for compensation, insisting that no causal relationship between the illness and factory effluent had been established. Instead the corporation pretended to be magnanimously helping the poor by making monetary "condolence gifts" to patients: ¥30,000 a year for a child, ¥100,000 a year for an adult, and ¥300,000 in the event of a death. Chisso seemed to be telling bereaved parents, often themselves suffering from the effects of mercury poisoning, that a child's life was worth a mere ¥300,000. Later, in court, this callous disregard for the dignity of life and human rights was roundly condemned as a "violation of public order and conscience."

Deliberate deception also occurred. As the number of Minamata-disease patients proliferated, the blue waters of the Shiranui Sea, into which Minamata Bay empties, were whitened with the upturned bellies of dead fish floating on the surface. The local fishers, impoverished by the depletion of the marine life on which they had depended, deluged Chisso with demands that the company stop pouring effluent into the sea. Aware that this would mean halting production, the company temporarily appeased the fishers by promising to install purification equipment. According to later court testimony by people working at the plant at the time, Chisso installed inferior equipment that did not remove the mercury that was causing the problem. Investment in the environment for the sake of respect for human life was sacrificed to the desire for greater production and profits.

Far too late, in 1968, the Ministry of Health and Welfare finally acknowledged that organic mercury in the effluent discharged by Chisso's Minamata plant was the cause of Minamata disease. But until then the company continued to pump poisonous wastes into the bay, causing almost a decade of needless human suffering and irreparably harming the environment.

By mid-1990, more than 900 people had died of Minamata disease. More than 2,000 patients had been certified, and another 3,000 were awaiting approval of their applications for certification. Altogether, the suffering brought about by massive environmental destruction had affected over 100,000 people, including unacknowledged victims. Chisso itself had been burdened with an enormous bill: ¥66 billion for compensation to patients and more than ¥16 billion for the installation of equipment to dispose of mercury-contaminated sludge. When interest is included, the company's tab was about ¥120 billion. Pleading financial hardship, Chisso had Kumamoto Prefecture issue bonds for payment of compensation, and the national government was compelled to act as guarantor. Of course, no amount of money can compensate for the loss of life and the destruction of the local community and natural environment. Minamata Bay, whose white sands and green pines once echoed to the voices of happy people gathering shellfish at low tide, is gone forever. Mercury-laden effluent has transformed the bay into a dead sea, much of which has now been filled in.

If only the Chisso executives had heeded the warning sounded by Hosokawa, if only they had acted in good faith at the outset, much of the damage could have been averted. Instead, they elected to follow a very different course. After forcing patients and their families to be satisfied with nominal "condolence gifts" and installing inferior purification equipment, at the end of 1959 they declared the Minamata-disease issue closed, hiding behind the smoke screen of these ineffectual measures. Thereupon Chisso actually stepped up production, in keeping with the government's policy of giving economic growth priority over all other considerations.

A number of noted scholars colluded with Chisso in trying to keep the lid on the Minamata-disease issue and thus helped enlarge the scope of the tragedy. They devised a number of unsubstantiated theories to hide the true cause of the disease. One scholar published a paper claiming that explosives dumped into the sea by the Imperial Navy at the end of World War II had corroded, releasing large quantities of toxic materials into the sea. These materials were alleged to have been ingested by fish and shellfish, which, when eaten, caused Minamata disease. This theory served the ends not only of Chisso but also of similar industries under the aegis of the Japan Chemical Industry Association and was therefore most welcome to the Ministry of

International Trade and Industry, overseer of Japan's industrial growth.

Another theory, concocted by a professor at a leading national university, was that the waters of Minamata Bay did not in fact have an especially high mercury content. He contended that waters in other regions contained comparable amounts of mercury without causing Minamata disease in the local inhabitants. This scholar insisted that it was not organic mercury but the presence of large quantities of toxic amines in the marine life of the Minamata area that caused the strange illness. But in measuring the mercury content of Minamata Bay, he tested only water from the upper levels of the bay, not the bottom mud in which the mercury was concentrated. A research team at the Kumamoto University School of Medicine, which had clearly established organic mercury as the cause as early as July 1959, criticized his methodology and dismissed his flawed theory as the result of inability to see the forest for the trees. Still another professor published a paper arguing that the people of the Minamata area fell ill because, being too poor to buy fresh fish, they ate older fish, which had a high toxic-amine content. Interestingly, at the end of the paper in which he proposed this theory, the professor thanked both Chisso and the JCIA for their cooperation with his research. A director of the JCIA requested the chairman of the Japan Association of Medical Sciences to form a committee to promote the theories of corroded explosives and toxic amines. This plot was foiled only because the JAMS chairman died, upon which the committee disbanded.

As soon as the Kumamoto University School of Medicine team identified the cause of the disease as organic mercury in factory effluent, Chisso leaped into action, claiming that its Minamata plant used inorganic mercury, not highly toxic organic mercury, in its production process and that because inorganic mercury cannot be converted into organic mercury (for so it was mistakenly believed at the time), Chisso's effluent could not be at fault.

It is true that certain scholars aided and abetted Chisso's attempt to evade responsibility. But even more telling was the attitude taken by the national newspapers. Endorsing the evasive position taken by the Ministry of Health and Welfare rather than the Kumamoto University data, they reported that the cause of the disease remained unknown. By doing so, in effect they sided with Chisso.

In presenting the theories of explosives and amines as "authoritative announcements," the newspapers behaved just as they had during World War II, when they uncritically published every pronouncement of Imperial Headquarters and in this way contributed to the expansion of the war. The press is supposed to lead society by creating informed public opinion. In this instance, however, at the crucial early stage public opinion was manipulated by biased "authoritative sources."

If even one national newspaper had realized the gravity of the Kumamoto University findings, investigated the problem, and mounted a campaign to do something about it, the power of public opinion throughout the nation would have halted the ravages of Minamata disease and many lives would have been saved. It might then have been possible to prevent economic growth from being given absolute priority and thus to avert some of the harm that has been done to our green isles. And the Japanese people might have avoided criticism by other nations as "economic animals" and despoilers of the global environment.

I wrote the Japanese version of this book in 1977, when the human and environmental tragedy of Minamata disease was still being played out, in an attempt to arouse a spirit of self-restraint and of atonement for what had been perpetrated at Minamata. From a global viewpoint, Minamata may be only a dot on the map. But the events there demonstrate all too clearly the disastrous consequences of neglecting antipollution measures and giving free rein to economic aggrandizement.

BITTER SEA

1. THE HEAVY BURDEN

O FF THE SHORES of Kumamoto Prefecture, on the west coast of Kyushu, the Shiranui Sea glowed deep blue in the dusk. Beyond an inky promontory, the flickering lights of the Amakusa Islands separated the dark of the land from the dark of the sky. Hand in hand with little Michiko Shiraishi, a blind, mad old woman with grossly swollen legs walked barefoot toward the dark sea. She sang in a cracked voice:

> "Throw down the heavy burden.
> The heavy burden is dirty.
> Away with it!
> Rip it up!
> What's useless should die.
> Tear the wadding from the padded clothes."

Michiko gazed up at this pathetic creature, her grandmother. Whenever the old woman crept out alone at night while the rest of the family slept, Michiko would leave her own bed to search for her. On winter nights she would find her grandmother standing in the falling snow, leaning on a length of green bamboo that served her as a walking stick. On one such occasion, struck by the solemnity of the old woman's appearance, her white head seeming to float in the darkness, Michiko drew near and called, "Grandma!"

"Is that you, Michiko?" the old woman replied. Letting go of her bamboo stick, she embraced the girl, who wept inexplicably as she pressed her face against the patched garment covering her grandmother's breast.

"Let's go home now," said Michiko as she picked up the bamboo stick and, taking the old woman's hand, started down the dark path beside the sea.

"Throw down the heavy burden. . . ." The old woman's soft singing was swallowed up in a solitude that muffled even the roar of the waves.

But Michiko was never able to do as the song said and throw down the heavy burden or abandon the useless. Like an incantation, her grandmother's murmured words settled deep in her heart and helped determine the fate that would lead her to devote herself to serving sufferers of the debilitating illness known as Minamata disease.

A mad old woman helped refine the compassion that Michiko felt for all injured life—a compassion that led her to take home wounded puppies and kittens and to share the family's meager food with wandering beggars. An encounter with a little war orphan, Tadeko, deepened her compassion still further.

Michiko's family was poor. The house they lived in was no more than a hovel that her father, Kametaro, had bought cheaply from a friend who had used it as a barn and tool shed. Michiko's grandfather Matsutaro had been a master carpenter of great talent and fame on the Amakusa Islands but had run up huge debts in connection with civil-engineering contracts. Kametaro had ruined the family trying to pay back his father's debts and had left Amakusa for Minamata, on the opposite side of the Shiranui Sea, less than four months after Michiko's birth in 1927. For a while the family had lived in Sakae-machi, near the center of the city, but eventually their house was seized for nonpayment of debts and they were forced to move to a poor settlement called Tonton Village, where they barely eked out a living.

After graduating from vocational school in Minamata at the age of sixteen, Michiko became a substitute teacher at a primary school in a neighboring town to help her family make ends meet, commuting by train. In those days schools did not pro-

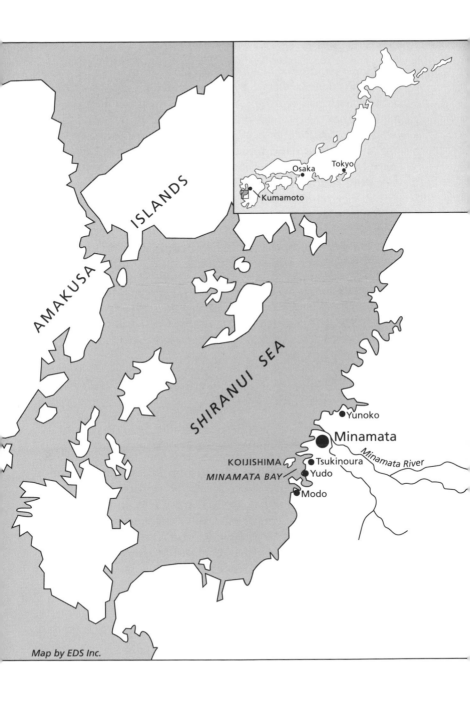

AMAKUSA

ISLANDS

SHIRANUI SEA

Osaka

Tokyo

Kumamoto

Yunoko

Minamata

KOIJISHIMA

Tsukinoura

Minamata River

MINAMATA BAY

Yudo

Modo

Map by EDS Inc.

vide lunch, and some children were too poor to bring their own. Her heart ached whenever she saw a child slip away at noon, embarrassed by having nothing to eat. Sometimes she gave these children her own lunch. Often she exhausted her salary buying school supplies for children who could not afford them or stopped off on her way to and from school to help a pupil's ailing parents. Later Michiko's mother, Haruno, said ruefully that though her daughter had gone to work to help the family, she spent all her money on other people and brought none of it home.

Even today, Michiko recalls her first meeting with Tadeko with sadness. It was shortly after World War II, when Michiko was working as a substitute teacher. Returning home from school on the train one spring evening, she spied a little girl, all skin and bones, huddled in the corner of a seat. The conductor said the child had boarded the train in Osaka, which had been leveled by American air raids, saying she wanted to go to her older sister in Kakogawa, Hyogo Prefecture. The rest of her family had been missing since the air raids. She had no ticket but refused to get off the train. She simply sat in the swaying train and stared blankly ahead. The sudden loss of her entire family had apparently robbed her of her senses.

Approaching the child, Michiko stretched out a hand to touch her dirty, unkempt hair. When she put a comb to it, she discovered it was infested with lice as big as sesame seeds. The thought of the uncertain fate awaiting the girl if she stayed on the train to Kagoshima City, on the southern tip of Kyushu, the end of the line, distressed Michiko so much that she decided to take the waif home with her.

The two of them got off the train at Minamata Station. Carrying Tadeko on her back, Michiko started the long walk to her house, which was at the mouth of the Minamata River. Stopping from time to time to rest and gaze up at the star-filled sky, she finally reached home.

The sudden appearance of a seriously ill child caused a flurry of activity. Her father ran to fetch a retired nurse who lived nearby, while her mother prepared some Chinese herbal medicine for the child's stomach and her grandfather split firewood to heat the bath. The blind grandmother stroked the little girl as Michiko's younger brothers and sister looked on with concern. Michiko herself prepared a thin rice gruel to feed the child.

Caring for Tadeko gave Michiko great satisfaction. Upon waking in the morning she ran to a neighboring field to pick fresh vegetables, and on her way home from school she bought fruit. On Saturday afternoons and Sundays she sat by the child's bed, showing her picture books or telling her stories. And when Tadeko's health improved, Michiko made clothes for her from whatever scraps of cloth she could find. The doctor at the nearby hospital, to which she frequently took the little girl, was so impressed by Michiko's selfless concern for an unknown child in such hard times that he refused to accept any payment for treatment or medicine.

Food was scarce, and Michiko's family, owning no farmland, was forced to subsist on government rice rations. There was barely enough for the family, let alone an outsider. Michiko made several trips to the city welfare office to arrange to have rations issued to Tadeko, as well. When she succeeded after ten days of effort, she was delighted at the thought that at last they could all live together with a measure of security.

When Tadeko was finally on her feet, Michiko occasionally took her to the seaside. They would climb a hill or a terraced field overlooking the sea and sit together, chin on knees, gazing out at the small spits of land that seemed to sleep peacefully in the gentle embrace of the sea.

At dusk, when the lights of the houses on the darkening mountains of the distant Amakusa Islands began to wink on, the Shiranui Sea sank into profound silence. In the morning, as the milky mists cleared away in the golden light, the blue expanse of the water flashed mirrorlike, and the gentle ripples on the surface lapped the green shores into waking.

Michiko thought of the sea as a cradle or as a mother. She felt that her life, like all other forms of life, was held in the embrace of the sea. On one of their seaside excursions, she turned to Tadeko, who was playing idly in the sand, and said, "Tadeko, I wonder why the sea is so gentle."

Although her physical health improved, Tadeko's mental state changed little. She remained withdrawn most of the time. Michiko's mother commented worriedly that the child never smiled. Tadeko's first expression of her own wishes took the form of a request to be allowed to go to her sister. This saddened Michiko, but her father said that clearly they could not live together indefinitely; soon it would be time to send the little girl away to her relatives.

Michiko knew Tadeko could not survive alone and longed to keep her. But nothing could alter Tadeko's desire to leave. The little girl smiled for the first time upon learning that she was about to be sent to her sister.

The time of parting arrived. Gazing up at the same starry sky that had hung over them a month and a half earlier when she had carried the child home on her back, Michiko walked hand in hand with Tadeko to Minamata Station, where the night train was waiting.

Michiko gave some soldiers who were on Tadeko's train a letter to the stationmaster at Kakogawa asking that he help the girl find her sister's house. Carrying the package of food and souvenirs Michiko had given her, Tadeko climbed aboard. The departure bell rang.

"Take care of yourself, Tadeko. We'll probably never meet again," said Michiko tearfully. Tadeko looked at her sadly. Michiko stood on the dark platform until the taillight of Tadeko's train disappeared into the night. Michiko never heard from Tadeko again.

Nineteen at the time and full of concern for the child, Michiko wrote an unpublished work, "Tadeko no Ki" (An Account of Tadeko). In this essay, naive and unformed though it is, can be detected the seeds of the writer of the acclaimed *Kugai Jodo: Waga Minamata-byo* (Paradise of the Bitter Sea: My Minamata Disease), an eloquent account of the sufferings of the victims of Minamata disease published in 1969.

Shortly after Tadeko's departure Michiko contracted tuberculosis and was confined to her home. As she lay in bed, she pondered the wartime educational system, which had extolled death for the sake of the nation. Feeling in some way personally responsible for the system, she resolved never to teach again and resigned her position.

A few years earlier Michiko had met a young man named Hiroshi Ishimure through her younger brother Hajime. Hiroshi's gentle personality impressed her, and she married him. Unable to find a good job, Hiroshi was working for a construction group. In addition to keeping the accounts, he was in charge of eleven laborers, including Hajime.

Though a laborer himself, Hiroshi was fond of reading. At the end of a long day's work he would often stop at a book shop on the way home and buy a volume or two with what little money he could spare. The local plant of Japan Nitrogen Fertilizer Company (Chisso, Japanese for "nitrogen," for short; the company was later renamed Chisso Corporation) was considered the best employer in Minamata, and Hiroshi's father wanted him to work there. But Hiroshi wanted to be a primary school teacher. While working on the construction team, he studied for the teacher's examination with Michiko's enthusiastic support. In the spring of 1947, not long after he and Michiko were married, he fulfilled his dream by passing the exam. But before leaving the construction group, he helped the eleven men who had worked under him find employment at the Chisso plant.

Soon Michiko was a mother. Since it was hard for the family to make ends meet on Hiroshi's meager salary, Michiko would strap her tiny son, Michio, to her back and join the ranks of black-market food barterers who traveled to rural areas in search of the food that was so scarce in the lean years following the war. She would obtain fish from the fishers of Minamata Bay and trade this for rice, sweet potatoes, and other produce. At Minamata Station, officials keenly scanned the incoming trains in search of female rice-runners. Michiko always put the rice she had obtained in a specially made bag, which she placed between the baby and her back, and walked by the officials with a nonchalant air.

Poor though they were, Michiko, Hiroshi, and their son lived in peace. Their happiest times were when, carrying bamboo baskets, the three of them went to Hachiman Beach, at the mouth of the Minamata River, to search for clams and the many other kinds of edible shellfish that could be found there. On holidays the white sands of the beach were thronged with families engaged in the same kind of hunt, and the happy voices of children rang through the blue-green pine groves nearby.

Hiroshi loved shellfish. It made Michiko happy to watch him devouring delicacies prepared from shellfish just gathered on the beach. He liked also to drink *shochu,* a strong distilled liquor made from rice or sweet potatoes, with his meals. When he got a little tipsy, he would burst into song, belting out his favorite ballads.

Michiko had been fond of literature since childhood. In the early years of her marriage she began writing verses in the traditional thirty-one-syllable *tanka* form. In 1953 she had her first verse published in *Hae* (South Wind), a journal for *tanka* poets that was published in Kumamoto Prefecture:

> If I go mad, like Grandma, I too
> May be kicked out of the house
> Bodily.

Works like this, delving into the dark recesses of the psyche, seemed out of place in the genteel magazine and jolted her associates, leaving them at a loss to evaluate her poetry. Gradually Michiko drifted away from *Hae,* which, with its concentration on the beauties of the seasons, its floral and natural themes, and its aversion to the painful aspects of humanity, began to strike her as superficially decorative.

Soon she took over the care of her mad grandmother, who had always been good to her. Before long, however, her grandmother died. Then Hajime killed himself by jumping in front of a train on his way home from a psychiatric hospital where he was undergoing treatment. As one member of her family after another died insane, Michiko began to fear that she too carried the seeds of insanity and even fancied that she was being controlled by the spirits of those whose injured lives had been cut short.

In 1954 Michiko met a local revolutionary poet, Gan Tanigawa, who began guiding her writing. He had quit his job on the copy desk of the *Nishi Nihon Shimbun* newspaper and joined the Japan Communist Party. A graduate of the elite University of Tokyo, he played a leading role in the party's prefectural committee.

The people of Minamata, whose literary heritage included two famous native sons, the brothers Soho Tokutomi and Roka Tokutomi, paid close attention to Gan Tanigawa and his older brother, Ken'ichi, a critic. They could not understand why Gan Tanigawa, graduate of a famous university and son of an ophthalmologist who was president of the Minamata Medical Association, should belong to the Communist Party.

Gan Tanigawa, notorious for his demanding nature, ruthlessly edited the poems Michiko showed him, in the process clarifying thoughts that had been only vaguely formed in her mind. She accepted all his changes without demur. Michiko was profoundly influenced by his advice to look directly at reality and to listen to the voice that rises from the depths of the psyche. Under his tutelage her writing gradually became more creative, and some of her poems were published in his mimeographed poetry journal *Chokusen* (Straight Line).

Around this time Tanigawa formed a literary circle of young people who met about once a week to discuss revolutionary literary and political topics. Michiko was an active and valued member of the group.

In July 1954 a patient suffering from a strange new illness was admitted to the hospital attached to the Chisso plant. Dr. Hajime Hosokawa, the hospital's director, realized immediately that he was being confronted with symptoms he had never seen before. He made a detailed record of all his observations on the patient's chart. The patient could not walk and had great difficulty articulating words, his sight and hearing were impaired, and he was emotionally unstable, vacillating between tears and laughter for no apparent reason. As time passed, his body began to be racked by violent convulsions. Despite Hosokawa's assiduous attention, the patient died a month after hospitalization.

When another patient with similar symptoms was admitted to the hospital in 1955, Hosokawa began to suspect that the number would increase still further. He was correct. On May 1, 1956, four patients suffering from what appeared to be a combination of epilepsy and palsy were admitted.

Tanigawa was in the same hospital at the time, undergoing treatment for a lung ailment. He too was under Hosokawa's care. One day Tanigawa received a visit from two close friends, Kaneyoshi Noda and Toshiyuki Kakita, both pediatricians. They told him of these new patients and of the difficulty they were having trying to treat them. The disorder, they said, resembled infantile paralysis in some respects. They feared that it was communicable and could become widespread. When Tanigawa asked whether they had reported this mysterious ailment to the public health authorities, they said they had been too preoccupied with treatment. "Well," said Tanigawa, "if you don't know what's causing it, you'd better report it or there'll be trouble later on."

Shortly after this, Hosokawa sent Noda to the public health office with the first official report on Minamata disease, as the syndrome came to be known. Impressed with the gravity of this report, the public health office, with the cooperation of the city government, the Minamata Medical Association, and Minamata Municipal Hospital, formed a committee to work out a strategy for dealing with the strange illness. When an investigative team visited Yudo, Tsukinoura, and Dezuki, the outlying districts from which the first patients had come, more and more victims were discovered. The fishing hamlets scattered along the coast of Minamata Bay were gripped by dread.

Tanigawa took a patient whose eyesight was severely impaired to see his father, who examined the fundus of the eye in Hosokawa's presence and found that the patient's field of vision was as restricted as if he were peering through a length of bamboo. Tanigawa's father said this was almost certainly caused by damage to the central nervous system.

After the examination Tanigawa and Hosokawa discussed the situation. Tanigawa said, "As the director of the company hospital, you're going to be in a tough position if it turns out that factory wastes are causing the problem. I hope you'll remain true to your conscience as a medical man." He sought to encourage the doctor by telling him about Henrik Ibsen's play *An Enemy of the People,* whose protagonist is a doctor who defies the authorities for the sake of the truth. Hosokawa replied firmly that he would do whatever he had to. The stern look on his face suggested that he was well aware how hard it would be to obey the dictates of his conscience in the face of big business. Later, when his experiments with effluent from the Minamata plant pitted him against Chisso's executives, he would fortify himself by reading Ibsen's play. He would then leave home for work with a letter of resignation in his pocket.

In 1958, before Minamata disease became a major social problem, Tanigawa left Minamata to take part in the labor disputes at the Miike coal mine of Mitsui Mining Company, near Omuta, Kumamoto Prefecture. While playing a leading role in this struggle, which helped pave the way for the 1960 movement opposing the Japan-U.S. security treaty, Tanigawa and some associates began publishing a magazine for circulation among sympathizers called *Saakuru Mura* (Circle Village). Several members of the Minamata literary group, including Michiko, contributed to the magazine. In fact, it was here that she published her first writings on Minamata disease.

✧

Because the strange new illness was at first thought to be communicable, some patients were quarantined in a special hospital for communicable diseases, Shirahama Hospital. Whenever a new patient was identified, white-coated public health inspectors hurried to his or her house to disinfect every nook and cranny. Having been cautioned against the danger of contagion, children held their breath as they passed houses reeking of disinfectant. Salespeople in stores put out specially labeled baskets in which patients' family members were required to place money when paying for purchases and from which they were to take their change. No one wanted to touch them.

Patients were also being admitted to the Chisso hospital, but soon it could no longer accommodate their growing number. Minamata Municipal Hospital set up a special ward for the most serious cases. For fear that rumors might cause anxiety among the general population, city officials instructed all hospital personnel to keep the ward's existence a secret.

In August 1956 the Kumamoto University School of Medicine sent a team to Minamata to investigate the situation and compile a report on the ailment. A copy of this document, which was treated as top secret, was sent to the Minamata city office. The report came to Michiko's attention when Satoru Akazaki, who worked in the city office and was a member of Tanigawa's literary circle, surreptitiously showed her a copy. The report documented patients' symptoms in detail from the onset of the illness to the time of death.

What Michiko saw was part of a volume that came to be called the Red Book because of the color of its cover. She was appalled at the suffering revealed. The dry data of the Red Book, her first contact with Minamata disease, had a powerful and lasting impact. Following is one of the case histories from this report.

Case #1: Fisher, 28, female.
Date of onset: July 13, 1956.
Major symptoms: Numbness of fingers; impaired hearing, speech, and consciousness; delirium.
Medical history: Robust health; no history of serious illness.
Family medical history: No obvious hereditary connection with present symptoms, but youngest brother (total of six siblings,

this one eight years old) contracted a similar nervous condition in May 1955.

Dietary habits: Normal.

Progress of disorder: July 13, numbness of the second, third, and fourth fingers of both hands. July 15, numbness in the area of the mouth, impaired hearing. July 18, inability to put on straw sandals easily, difficulty in walking. Starting about the same time, impaired speech, tremors of the fingers, occasional jerky involuntary movements of the kind associated with chorea [a disorder of the nervous system characterized by irregular jerking movements caused by involuntary muscular contractions]. In August, further difficulty in walking. August 7, patient admitted to Shirahama Hospital, Minamata. The following day, chorea becomes violent and is accompanied by ballismus [violent flinging movements of the limbs]. Patient is delirious and occasionally howls like a dog. Though sedatives induce sleep, involuntary movements of the limbs persist. These symptoms continue until August 26. Inability to eat normally induces severe debility. Involuntary movements abate somewhat. Temperature normal from onset of illness until August 26, when patient begins to run a fever of 38 degrees Celsius [100.4 degrees Fahrenheit]. Patient admitted to this department August 30.

Findings of examination at time of admission to this department: Slight frame. Extreme debility. Total loss of consciousness. Face severely wizened. At roughly one-minute intervals, face stiffens in an expression of agony. Howls with mouth open wide. No words. At the same time, limbs racked with movements characteristic of chorea and ballismus. Torso stiffens and arches backward. Temperature 38 degrees C. Pulse 105, rapid and feeble. Poor muscular tension. Pupils contracted. Pupils' response to light a little slow.

Record following admission to this department: Nasal feeding initiated August 31. Involuntary movements continue August 31 but abate September 1. Muscular flaccidity; no response when limbs touched. Temperature 39 degrees C [102.2 degrees F], pulse 122, respiration 33. General condition worse. Involuntary movements resume about 2:00 A.M. September 2. Condition develops into delirium accompanied by howling. This continues until phenobarbital administered by injection. Patient subsides and falls asleep about 10:00 A.M. At 10:00 P.M. pulse 120, respiration 56, blood pressure 160 over 70. Death at 3:35 A.M. September 3.

The realization that this appalling illness was attacking people in Minamata, her home, made Michiko tremble uncontrollably. But she immediately began to reflect on suspicious events over the past few years. She recalled newspaper accounts of dead mullet found floating in Minamata and Fukuro bays. Later reports of cats in the Yudo and Modo districts dashing about madly and throwing themselves into the sea had prompted a fleeting premonition that human beings might also be in peril. Now, in the Red Book, she saw her fears confirmed.

In 1958 Michiko's son, Michio, contracted tuberculosis and was admitted to Minamata Municipal Hospital. By an odd turn of fate, his ward was next to the special ward housing twenty Minamata-disease patients. The Red Book fresh in her memory, Michiko found herself drawn inexorably to their ward. On her very first visit, she heard the eerie doglike howling she had read about and saw countless fingernail scratches scoring the white walls of the new ward.

Michiko describes her initial encounter with the patients, which transformed her life, in *Paradise of the Bitter Sea:*

Toward the end of May 1959—far too late—I visited one of the patients, Yuki Sakagami. Born in 1915, she was from the Tsukinoura district of Minamata. She was the thirty-seventh person identified as suffering from the baffling disease.

May is a fresh, fragrant month in Minamata. Yuki's second-floor window looked out on the deep, clear green of the mountains and the gently curving course of the Minamata River, along whose banks stretched fields of ripening wheat and broad beans still in flower. The air seemed to shimmer through a veil of heat.

On the way to her room I encountered a number of other patients. I cannot say I actually met them, since most were unconscious. Those who clung to awareness merely stared with dilated, unblinking eyes at the death that was about to consume them. They seemed poised on the brink of death, uncertain whether to advance or retreat.

Tsurumatsu Kama, one of these dying people, had fallen from his bed and lay face up on the floor. Born in 1903 and a fisher from Komenotsu in the city of Izumi, he was the eighty-second patient to be identified. He died in 1960. He was a handsome man, with a clean-cut jaw, high-bridged nose, finely molded brow, and piercing eyes. Although his cheeks twitched spasmodically from time to time, they still showed traces of ruddy color. But his arms and legs were like sticks of driftwood stripped to the grain by the waves, the wind-burned skin stretched taut over the bones. The lingering tan of his face was vivid testimony to the speed with which death was approaching.

The medical records describe patients rendered inarticulate by mercury poisoning as howling like dogs. These howls, high-pitched or deep and throaty, forced out with the last remnant of physical strength, reverberated through the corridor. They transformed the ward, despite its sparkling newness and the shimmering early-summer light spilling in from the windows, into a dark, dank cave.

I found myself slowing as I approached Tsurumatsu Kama's room. I did not immediately take in all the details of his appearance, especially the fierce look in his eyes, as he lay on the floor. But as I began to walk slowly past his half-open door, I was brought to a halt by a vivid sensation of breath swirling around my feet and took a closer look. The living often delude themselves that the dead rest in peace. But the eyes of this dying man told me that his spirit had no intention of giving in to death without a fight.

That encounter prompted me to ask myself whether I could bear to spend the rest of my life as nothing but a humble housewife living along the lower reaches of the Minamata

River, gazing at the sea and murmuring poems to the crabs on the beach. I was filled with self-loathing. Tsurumatsu Kama's sad eyes, driftwood limbs, and stubborn refusal to die quietly took possession of my spirit.

Michiko walked on to the next room in a daze. There she saw a patient convulsed in a grotesque dance, arms and legs raised rigidly toward the ceiling. Michiko fell to the floor, collapsing under the shock of the emotions aroused by what she was seeing. The unspeakable misery of these people burned itself into her mind, and she felt herself being helplessly sucked into an abyss of despair.

Though she herself was so frail that she seemed on the edge of death, she resolved to devote whatever life remained to her to lifting the heavy veil concealing the hellish world of Minamata-disease victims by writing about their condition, in the hope that someday the world would pay attention and come to their aid. Her decision was not prompted by a sense of duty; her motivation was, rather, that of one determined to leave a last testament before dying. This woman, who had been unable to see a suffering child without offering help, was about to embark on a struggle in behalf of the innocent victims of Minamata disease. Convinced that never had human dignity been so grossly violated, she was spurred to battle by a mixture of compassion and anger. The spirits of the patients possessing her were her guides through a hell echoing with the words of her demented grandmother: "Throw down the heavy burden." Michiko could not escape this hell; the burden she bore was heavy indeed.

2. INTO THE ABYSS

IN JULY 1959 a team from the Kumamoto University School of Medicine, after considering magnesium, selenium, thallium, and dozens of other substances, determined that the strange illness was caused by organic mercury entering the sea in waste discharged from the Chisso plant in Minamata.

Chisso used large quantities of mercury as a catalyst in the production of vinyl chlorides and acetaldehyde. The Kumamoto University team found that so much of the substance had been pumped out with factory waste that the concentration of mercury was two kilograms per ton of effluent at Hyakken Harbor. On the basis of data supplied by Chisso, the team calculated that six hundred tons of mercury had already been poured into the sea. Ingested by fish and shellfish, it attacked the nervous systems of people who ate this seafood. Chisso, however, tried vigorously to discredit this explanation, insisting that only harmless inorganic mercury was used in its production processes and erroneously claiming that inorganic mercury could not change into poisonous organic mercury.

At that time Akazaki was working in the Hygiene Department of the Minamata city office. Doctors from Kumamoto University were examining victims of mercury poisoning at Minamata Municipal Hospital and in the fishing communities in and around the city. It was Akazaki's job to take patients to the hospital or to take the doctors to patients' homes in a microbus on days when the university doctors were examining patients.

Consequently, he knew more than almost anyone else about the true conditions of the patients.

In January 1960 Michiko published an article titled "Kibyo" (Strange Illness) in *Circle Village*. Until then, people had been too afraid of Chisso to write directly about the misery of those afflicted. Akazaki and others connected with the literary group publishing the magazine were surprised and a little apprehensive when this unknown housewife wrote boldly about events taking place right under their noses in Minamata. But most residents, aware that the city's prosperity depended on Chisso, were cool to Michiko's charges.

Learning that Michiko had resolved to delve even more deeply into the problem, Akazaki felt obliged to help her. He disagreed with the city officials' policy of currying favor with Chisso by attempting to conceal the existence of the illness and thus keep it from becoming a major social problem. As a civil servant, he also felt that playing down this strange new disorder and ignoring those who needed help was a violation of the duty of local government. Instead of trying to cover up the illness, he believed, the city should offer willing assistance to those suffering from it. He saw no conflict with his duty as a public employee in revealing the patients' true conditions to Michiko, believing that the city government had no grounds for prosecuting him as long as he did not violate the national law governing local-government employees.

At the same time, he was aware that this attitude was unrealistic. In a city like Minamata, which was in thrall to Chisso, criticism of the company would inevitably lead to persecution and slander. But as long as Michiko was determined to concern herself with the sickness, he felt compelled to cooperate, though he realized it meant the end of all hope of promotion. Even so, he often lay awake at night wondering why he had chosen to challenge the Establishment when there were much easier ways to live.

Akazaki, like Michiko, felt compassion for all injured life. His oldest daughter had been stricken with infantile paralysis at the age of two and could barely walk even with the aid of crutches.

Sometimes, when he had drunk a little too much sakè, he would weep at the thought of what would become of his daughter when she reached womanhood. Her life, too, was injured. In that she could never recover from her paralysis, she was like those children born with Minamata disease. Whenever he saw such a child he was reminded of his own daughter.

The victims of Minamata disease kept very much to themselves, avoiding strangers. Because of his job, however, Akazaki had to learn as much as he could about their circumstances and visited their homes almost daily. At first they fell silent when he approached. But whenever the fishers held a get-together, he would take along a bottle and join them, drinking sakè from a teacup and chatting. Gradually the fishers accepted him. "At first we thought you were an outsider, Mr. Akazaki, because you're from city hall, but now we see you're really just like us." Once trust had been established, members of patients' families freely discussed their troubles with him. In time even some of the patients themselves, whose hearts had been tightly closed to outsiders, began to relax in his presence.

Whenever doctors from Kumamoto University or from the Minamata public health office were scheduled to examine patients at home, Akazaki would phone Michiko and ask her to go along. In her dark blue kimono and worn-down wooden clogs, she would hop on her bicycle and dash off to the city office, where she would join the party of doctors and nonchalantly board the city microbus.

Michiko accompanied the doctors into the patients' houses, where conditions were often appalling. In dark rooms reeking of ordure, the wasted and lice-infested patients lay on thin pallets spread on tattered tatami mats and surrounded by torn shoji panels. Sitting unobtrusively in a corner, Michiko listened to the patients' complaints and jotted down an occasional note. Both doctors and patients assumed she was a nurse from the public health office.

Akazaki always asked Michiko to go with him when he visited patients on his own, too. On these occasions, ignoring the fleas that hopped onto her kimono, she drew near the patients and listened carefully to everything they said. She tried to make them more comfortable, but there was nothing she could do when they were seized by convulsions and thrashed from one side of the room to the other.

When a family's major provider was stricken, income ceased, and it became very difficult to make ends meet. Nonetheless, the patients' families received no financial aid at all. Michiko angrily asked Akazaki why the city did nothing to help these poor people. The reply was that most families still possessed boats, which were considered assets and thus disqualified them from receiving public aid.

Michiko was enraged to learn that city officials were hiding behind the letter of the law although they knew that the fishers no longer had safe waters in which to fish and that their boats were rotting on the shore. Once, speaking loudly enough for Akazaki to hear, she reassured a patient, "Everything will be all right. Mr. Akazaki works in the city office, but he's an understanding person. He'll see that you get the help you need. Till then, just try to take it easy."

All too aware of the heartless policies of the city officials, Akazaki was as upset as if he himself were at fault. As a humble civil servant, he could not talk out of turn. But this made no difference to Michiko, who for the patients' sake would say things that sent chills up his spine. When she suggested that they distribute leaflets describing the suffering that victims of Minamata disease were being forced to endure because of Chisso, he recoiled in horror. Open combat with the company could only result in their ostracism. Sometimes he detested himself for being so much more timid than Michiko, who was willing to do battle with mighty Chisso to help the sick. Watching her toss her bobbed hair in anger, indifferent to public opinion, desiring nothing for herself and willing to lie down beside the patients in their hovels, Akazaki would renew his own determination.

Sometimes it was already evening when they left the city office to visit patients. The spiritual bond between them deepened as they talked together, gazing at the lights of the Amakusa Islands twinkling across the Shiranui Sea. Often they became so engrossed in conversation that they missed the last bus and did not reach home till after midnight. Still upset by the suffering they had seen, they would walk the several kilometers to the city, talking all the while. Michiko would speak of the way these humble folk had lived in peace, relying on the calm Shiranui Sea—once their sustenance but now the source of death and destruction. She talked about the way they were compelled to watch their loved ones die and then to see their own bodies ravaged by this mysterious disease. Sometimes they would duck beneath the awning of a street stand for a drink of sakè to try to ease the impact of what they had witnessed, but they could not erase the memory of the patients' twisted faces.

Many of these people had crossed to Minamata from the Amakusa Islands, drawn by the dream of a better life. Michiko wrote about them as follows:

> The people of Amakusa call Minamata "the other shore." When rumors that a factory was going to be built on the other shore reached Amakusa, many residents started thinking about moving to Minamata. A plant there would mean they could probably find work without having to move too far from their homes and families. The likelihood that a plant would also turn Minamata into an important city made the prospect of crossing over all the more attractive. Growing numbers of people moved to Minamata.
>
> Though few of them had any desire to work at the Chisso plant, they felt that even living on the city's periphery, like oysters and barnacles clinging to rocks in the sea, would make them part of a cosmopolitan scene. And although they themselves did not work for Chisso, they took pride in the plant as it grew larger and more imposing. They would gaze at it proudly from their boats when they were out fishing.

And whenever they came across fishing boats from Amakusa, they would boast of how strong Minamata's economy was and of the important work the plant was doing.

Most of these people belonged to fishing families living on the fringe of society. Natives of Minamata referred to them condescendingly as "those people from Amakusa." But though they reaped no real benefit from the city's growth, I believe they were more deeply attached to Minamata than many other citizens. These were the good-natured people who became the victims of Minamata disease.

Susumu Sugimoto, who headed a fishing group in the hamlet of Modo, was one such person. Since most of the patients were fishers and their families, Michiko realized that to write about them intelligently she would have to learn about their work. Feeling that the head of a fishing group would be a good source of information, one summer day in 1959 she climbed the hill to Sugimoto's house. She could see all the way to the Amakusa Islands. A small boat gliding across the mirrorlike waters of Modo Bay left a faint wake. She knew nothing about Sugimoto's family; she was unaware that his wife was gravely ill with Minamata disease and that he himself had been stricken.

Born around the turn of the century, Sugimoto had fished the Shiranui Sea as long as he could remember. Fishing was his life, and he was far and away the best fisher in the community. He could tell whether the fishing would be good or bad on any given day. If he advised putting the nets away and staying home, boats that did venture forth were certain to return empty except for their grumbling crews. If he said, "There'll be a big catch today," there would be. His intuition was uncanny. He understood fish so well that he seemed to know the direction they would take. Though he never watched the televised weather forecasts, he predicted the winds and other meteorological phenomena with uncanny accuracy.

Sugimoto was proud of his skills. He was also proud of his only daughter, Eiko, whom he had brought up to be a good fisher and who went fishing with him even when her wedding was drawing near. He and his daughter were famous for their close bond. Eiko, too, was happiest out on the waters of the Shiranui Sea, fishing with her father.

When Michiko first visited Sugimoto, mercury poisoning had already attacked his once-hardy body. Gazing out the window at the deep blue expanse of the sea, he said wistfully, "I'd like to go out just once more."

Though he was a taciturn man who rarely talked to anyone but fellow fishers to whom he was especially close, for some reason he readily told Michiko everything he knew about fishing in the Shiranui Sea. A real fisher has to be able to spot schools of small sardines skimming the waves like pine needles flying in the wind, he told her, because deep below the little fish are the big ones. No mention was made of Michiko's writing a book, but the will driving her to compose a "last testament" on Minamata disease must have conveyed itself to him. In telling her of the bygone days when the fishing had been rich and good, he too may have been pronouncing a kind of last testament.

Sugimoto was the forty-fourth person to die of the disease. Eiko carried on her father's work, but eventually she also succumbed.

Minamata Bay had always been famous for the abundance and variety of its fish. The current of the Shiranui Sea parts to flow around the island of Koijishima, situated at the mouth of the bay. Uniting again beyond the island, the current flows into the bay. Fish from these waters were praised as especially delicious. Borne on the current, they entered the bay, where there was plenty of food. Great schools of sea bream, gray mullet, and other fish swam in the depths, and shoals of sardines rippled the surface of the waters. The local fishers took what they wanted from this abundance and felt themselves blessed. They desired no further riches.

It was into this treasure-trove of sea life that the toxic wastes of the Chisso plant were steadily being emptied. Suddenly the number of fish dropped drastically. Sometimes the surface of the bay was covered with the floating bodies of dead mullet. Five years after the initial outbreak of Minamata disease, catches were less than one-tenth the size they had been, and the few fish that were caught were branded as contaminated. Local fish dealers agreed not to purchase them, and thus effectively excluded them from the market. Citizens replaced the fish in their diet with meat and canned food. Useless fishing boats were hauled up on beaches and left to rot.

The fishers could only gaze helplessly at their dying sea. Observing them, Michiko had an uneasy premonition that in their frustration they were going to cause serious trouble. Unlike the men who fish the rough open seas, the fishers of the gentle Shiranui Sea rarely show anger. Most are shy and reserved. But not even the mildest-mannered people can be expected to wait docilely for death when their livelihood has been snatched from them and they have no idea where their next meal is coming from.

In August 1959 the Minamata Fishermen's Cooperative declared that effluent from the Chisso plant was ruining their fishing and demanded compensation of ¥100 million. About three hundred demonstrators, carrying banners and placards and yelling that Chisso was trying to destroy the fishers, marched through the city and pushed their way into the plant, where they demanded that the plant manager acknowledge Chisso's responsibility for the pollution.

Claiming that no causal relationship between the plant's effluent and Minamata disease had been established, Chisso flatly refused the fishers' demand. Undaunted, they tried again. This time the company offered a "consolation payment" of ¥3 million. But the fishers were unwilling to be bought off so cheaply. They demanded full compensation for the damage done to their fishing grounds, but Chisso would not listen.

Later, in collective bargaining, Chisso made an offer of ¥10 million, a sum eventually raised to a "final offer" of ¥13 million. At that point the talks broke down. The fishers waiting outside the plant were so enraged by the company's highhanded attitude that they forced their way into the building, breaking down the door and smashing windows. Police were called to disperse them. Taken aback by their first encounter with the police, the fishers suppressed their anger and departed quietly.

Through the efforts of Todomu Nakamura, the mayor of Minamata, and a member of the prefectural assembly who had once belonged to the plant's labor union the two sides finally agreed that Chisso would make a payment of ¥35 million. Although this amounted to less than ¥117,000 for each of the three hundred fishing families affected, the fishers were compelled to accept the offer when the arbitrators warned that because of the Chisso plant's importance to Minamata further protests would earn them the animosity of the entire citizenry. This brought the roughly month-long fishers' struggle to an end.

Meanwhile, effluent continued to pour into the sea.

3. CORPORATE CHICANERY

ORIGINALLY, Chisso had pumped wastes into Hyakken Harbor, to the south of the Minamata plant. In September 1958, however, as pollution grew increasingly severe and the damage to the fishing industry steadily more serious, the company began secretly pumping wastes into the mouth of the Minamata River, to the north, instead. Hosokawa requested Chisso executives to put a stop to this practice, since it showed a reckless disregard for human life and was bound to endanger still more people, but his plea was ignored.

The doctor's fears proved prophetic. In 1959 the toxic effects of organic-mercury pollution began appearing as far north of Minamata as Ashikita, fifteen kilometers away. Dead fish were found floating on the surface of the water, and cats began dying in convulsions. Hachiman Beach, where Michiko and her family had once happily gathered shellfish, was ruined. The white bellies of dead fish dotted the water. The stench of rotting fish and shellfish, mingled with the noisome fumes of factory effluent, hung in the air like a miasma.

Not long after Michiko's initial visit to the special ward for Minamata-disease patients in Minamata Municipal Hospital, people living in Hachiman and Funatsu, near the new outlet, began exhibiting the symptoms of what they had half-jokingly called the "dancing-cat disease," till then concentrated in southern communities, such as Yudo and Modo.

When the extent of the pollution became apparent, Chisso

closed the northern outlet. But the damage done to the fishing industry sparked protests from fishermen's cooperatives throughout the Shiranui Sea coastal area—just when Chisso seemed to have triumphed in its struggle with the Minamata cooperative.

On November 2, 1959, the National Diet sent an investigative commission to Minamata. About four thousand fishers and sympathizers, including Michiko, gathered in the street in front of Minamata Municipal Hospital to march to the Chisso plant, where they were to conduct a rally and petition the commission for help. Some demonstrators carried huge banners bearing the slogans "Give us back our beautiful Shiranui Sea!" and "Stop factory wastes that kill the sea!" Voices arose from the crowd as it made its way to the plant: "We were born on these shores, but now they've been turned into a hell. Please use your political influence to save us!"

The marchers stopped in front of the plant's main gate. Suddenly a woman stepped from the crowd. Advancing toward the commission members, who were standing in front of the plant, she cried out, "Please hear what we have to say! You Diet members are like mothers and fathers to us!" At these impassioned words a hush fell over the gathering. The woman continued: "We are honored to petition you, people we would ordinarily never be able to meet. We have lost our children to Minamata disease. Our husbands are out of work because there are no fish to catch. And even if there were fish, no one would buy them from us. So far we've blamed it all on bad luck and gritted our teeth. But we've come to the end of our tether. We can't take any more. Please have mercy and help us." Michiko saw that the commission members were listening attentively.

The fishers then asked the officials of the Chisso plant to agree to group negotiations but were refused. At this point what had been a peaceful demonstration was transformed into an angry mob rushing toward the factory. The main gate, tightly barred and topped with barbed wire, was guarded by riot police. Enraged by Chisso's use of police to thwart them, those in the forefront of the crowd shouted, "Send somebody out to talk to us! Send out the top boss!"

Still calling out wildly, some of the demonstrators climbed over the gate and opened it from within. Mayhem ensued. Adding machines were smashed. Teletype equipment sailed through the air. Office supplies were dumped into the hated factory-waste conduit. Over a hundred people, on both sides, were injured.

Legal proceedings brought against the fishers by Chisso had aggravated their anger. In mid-October the Kumamoto Prefecture Federation of Fishermen's Cooperatives had sponsored a protest rally. On that occasion about seven hundred people crowded into the grounds of the Minamata plant, demanding a halt to pollution of the sea. When they were rebuffed, the fishers forced their way into the main building, smashing windows and injuring a guard. Chisso submitted a complaint to the Minamata police accusing a number of demonstrators of violence. The police immediately initiated an investigation and eventually made several arrests. The local fishers were hardly able to contain their anger over this incident. The sight of police guarding the plant again on November 2 seemed proof of complicity between the company and the police.

But much of the local population resented the fishers, since halting pollution would mean curtailing Chisso's production. Not only the Chisso labor union, which had a natural interest in the plant's profitability, but also the Chamber of Commerce and Industry, women's groups, and many other organizations in Minamata regarded the fishers with hostility.

The fishers of the Shiranui Sea were surrounded by foes. To Michiko, observing them on November 2, they seemed flayed so raw by mental and material anguish that the slightest touch could sting them into action. In her opinion, only the sloth of a public administration that winked at the responsibility of the business enterprise causing the problem and ignored the plight of the fishing population and the suffering of the disease victims could have driven these gentle people to violence. She felt that an administration that made no serious attempt to combat the disease or help its victims but strove only to serve the capitalist enterprise behind the disease symbolized the nation's abandonment of its own people.

The fishermen's cooperatives along the Shiranui Sea had calculated that the damage to their industry amounted to ¥2.5 billion. Kumamoto Prefecture Governor Kosaku Teramoto, Minamata Mayor Todomu Nakamura, and the other members of the arbitration council, however, had worked out their own figures. They proposed paying the fishers a lump sum of ¥35 million and financing a recovery fund of ¥65 million. But ¥10 million in damages for the November 2 break-in was to be subtracted from the ¥35 million payment; and since the recovery fund amounted to a loan from the company, the fishers would actually receive only ¥25 million, a mere 1 percent of the damages calculated by the cooperatives. Divided among the seven thousand fishing families on the Shiranui Sea coast, this would give each family just over ¥3,500—less than $10 (at the time the dollar was worth ¥360). This was all the compensation they were to receive for the loss of their fishing grounds. In response to the fishers' other demand, that the plant stop polluting the sea, Chisso said it was installing purification equipment. With these steps the fishers were silenced.

Lack of concern for the welfare of ordinary people was also reflected in the paltry compensation offered to Minamata-disease patients at the end of 1959. Although overshadowed by the uproar caused by the local fishers, in the summer of 1959 patients began agitating for compensation for the irreversible harm done to their health. On November 28 the Mutual Aid Association of the Families of Minamata Disease Patients, which had been founded in August 1958 and now had about fifty members, began a sit-in in front of the Chisso plant's main gate to support its demand for compensation of ¥3 million per patient. That evening the thirtieth death from Minamata disease was announced: a forty-six-year-old fisher from Ashikita. Toxic waste from the Minamata River outlet had claimed its first victim.

Many city folk cast cold looks and even stones at the those taking part in the sit-in, accusing them of ingratitude for opposing the plant on which Minamata's prosperity depended. No matter that its wastes had polluted the Shiranui Sea and caused many deaths; Minamata still crouched in deference before the citadel of Chisso.

The patients, isolated and shunned, began to despair as the sit-in dragged on. The fishers at least had settled their dispute, albeit for a pittance. Having already sold all their valuables and exhausted every avenue for loans, most of the patients' families could barely scrape together enough money for food. The end of the year was approaching, but none of them would be able to buy the traditional seasonal treats. They grew impatient and edgy but persevered grimly, though their only shelter from the cold December winds was a tent borrowed from the plant's labor union. But human beings can be colder than the north wind, as the union soon revealed by demanding the return of its tent. The demonstrators washed the tent before returning it.

Chisso continued to ignore them, and finally they felt compelled to turn for help to the mayor and the governor, who had helped negotiate the settlement with the fishermen's cooperatives. A negotiating committee of five was set up, including Governor Teramoto, Mayor Nakamura, and Yutaka Iwao, chairman of the prefectural assembly. Having already forced a meager settlement on the fishers, these men could hardly be expected to have the interests of the patients at heart. But because of their previous experience, they seemed the only people qualified to deal with Chisso. From the outset it was apparent that negotiations would follow company dictates. But after a month-long sit-in the demonstrators, by now mentally and physically exhausted, were ready to clutch at any straw.

The patients were offered the following sums: ¥30,000 a year for a child, ¥100,000 a year for an adult, and ¥300,000 in the event of a death. Making the most of the patients' weak position, Chisso demonstrated a condescending compassion, saying, in effect, "Since it has not been proved that the plant's effluent is the cause of Minamata disease, these payments are not compensation but 'condolence gifts' offered in sympathy." The company also forced the victims to sign an agreement including the following provision: "Even should it be proved at some future date that factory effluent is the cause of Minamata disease, the recipients agree to make no further demand for compensation."

When the patients' representatives hesitated to accept these terms, they were warned repeatedly by Mayor Nakamura and other members of the committee that if they refused this offer the committee would wash its hands of the affair. In other words, they could either accept the compensation offered or expect to get nothing at all. Confronted with this choice and afraid that they would indeed get nothing, the representatives handed over their seals and watched as they were stamped on the written agreement to signify compliance.

The agreement was concluded on December 30. With that, a dark curtain of apparent finality fell over the victims and the entire problem of Minamata disease.

Hosokawa, the first person to detect cases of Minamata disease, suspected that effluent from the Chisso plant was to blame. In July 1959 he began to test his hypothesis by sprinkling polluted water on food fed to a number of cats. On October 7 one of the cats, labeled number 400, began to exhibit the same symptoms seen in human victims of the disease. After performing an autopsy on the animal on November 24, he sent samples of brain tissue to the pathology laboratory of Kyushu University for analysis. The tissue demonstrated the loss of cerebellum cells characteristic of Minamata disease. Hosokawa immediately reported the results to Chisso. On November 30 he received orders to stop his experiments. The remaining cats were secretly destroyed.

Hosokawa's direct appeal to Kiichi Yoshioka, president of Chisso, and other top executives for permission to continue his experiments and share his findings with the outside world was rejected. In 1962 he resigned from Chisso, and later he developed lung cancer. But in 1970, during the first trial that grew out of the Minamata problem, he testified from his hospital bed that as a physician he wanted to make two things clear: first, cat 400 had definitely demonstrated symptoms of Minamata disease; and second, his recommendation that the Minamata plant's waste outlet not be switched from Hyakken Harbor to the mouth of the Minamata River, since doing so was tantamount to irresponsibly experimenting with human lives, had been ignored. He died later that year.

The doctor's testimony makes it abundantly clear that Chisso was fully aware that its plant's effluent was responsible for Minamata disease at the time that company representatives were negotiating with patients and coercing them into accepting "condolence gifts" on the pretext that no causal relation had been established. That is why Chisso, clearly realizing that its pollutants were in fact to blame, insisted that the patients agree to relinquish all future claims against the company.

This was not the full extent of Chisso's perfidy. The purification equipment Chisso had told the fishermen's cooperatives it was installing at a cost of ¥60 million was completed in December 1959. Addressing the local dignitaries invited to a ceremony celebrating the installation of the equipment, Chisso President Yoshioka boasted, "The waste water from our plant is now as clean as the water in the Minamata River." He then filled a glass with water from a drainage pipe and drank it down.

However, the all-important pipes carrying off wastes from the acetaldehyde production process were not connected to the purification equipment, as people working in the plant at the time later testified in court. For almost ten years after the discovery that cat 400 demonstrated Minamata-disease symptoms, Chisso continued to pump mercury-laden wastes into the sea at a rate of five hundred tons an hour. By the time the government officially recognized the causal relation between the plant's effluent and the disease in 1968, many more people had died.

In Michiko's eyes, refusing to listen to Hosokawa and thereby causing unnecessary deaths was equivalent to deliberate poisoning. Had Chisso heeded the doctor's warning, admitted that organic mercury was the cause of the problem, and taken steps to rectify the situation, it might have been possible to avert the outbreak in the mid-1960s of the same symptoms in Niigata Prefecture, northern Honshu, caused by organic mercury discharged into the Agano River by the chemicals manufacturer Showa Denko.

✧

A number of specious theories were concocted to deceive the public and divert attention from the true cause of Minamata disease. Takeji Oshima, managing director of the authoritative Japan Chemical Industry Association, claimed that at the end of World War II the Imperial Navy had dumped large quantities of explosives into Fukuro Bay, south of Minamata, and that with the passage of time the casings had corroded, permitting toxic substances to leak into the water. These, he argued, were the true cause of Minamata disease.

Even though a research team from Kumamoto University had already thoroughly discredited this theory, the JCIA resurrected it because if organic mercury were accepted as the causal agent not only Chisso but also many other companies under the JCIA's aegis would be in trouble. The Ministry of International Trade and Industry, whose main concern was the protection of Japanese industry, is said to have been relieved when the press credulously reported the corroded-explosives theory as if it were fact.

Another false theory, that of toxic amines, was the brainchild of Professor Raisaku Kiyoura of the Tokyo Institute of Technology. Claiming that the level of organic mercury in Minamata Bay was not significantly higher than the level in other bays and that mercury-contaminated fish were found in other regions where the disease did not manifest itself, Kiyoura argued that organic mercury could not be the cause of Minamata disease. He claimed that the true villain was toxic amines in fish and shellfish. But Kiyoura had tested water taken only from the upper levels of Minamata Bay, where concentrations of mercury were relatively low, whereas the real problem lay in the high concentration of mercury in the bottom mud. The Kumamoto University research team criticized Kiyoura's slipshod methodology and condemned his theory as a classic case of inability to see the forest for the trees.

Endorsing Kiyoura's theory, Professor Kikuji Tokita of Toho University advanced the droll idea that poor fisherfolk fell victim to Minamata disease because they could afford to eat only the leftover fish from the catches they took to market. This practice was dangerous, he said, because the concentration of toxic amines is highest in fish that has begun to spoil. Tokita's paper expounding this theory, which is said to have been compiled with MITI's cooperation, thanks both the JCIA and Chisso for assisting his research.

In an attempt to discredit Kumamoto University's findings, the JCIA established the so-called Tamiya Committee, headed by Takeo Tamiya, chairman of the Japan Association of Medical Sciences, to promote the corroded-explosives and toxic-amines theories. Unfortunately for the JCIA, Tamiya died not long afterward and the committee disbanded.

Behind these schemes Michiko saw Chisso's money and power manipulating compliant scientists. But the ultimate culprit, in her eyes, was a government willing to sacrifice its people to production and economic growth for the sake of gaining a place among the leading industrial nations of the world. Chisso's cavalier treatment of Minamata-disease patients was condoned because it was in keeping with the prevailing attitude that business takes precedence over everything else, even human life.

Having apparently placated both the fishers and the patients, Chisso and the Minamata municipal authorities worked together to persuade the public that the affair was over and done with. The extent to which Chisso dominated the city and was thus able to impose a taboo on the Minamata-disease issue is revealed by municipal tax revenue statistics for 1961. The majority of the city's fifty thousand inhabitants depended on Chisso for a living, and fully half of the total tax revenue of ¥230 million was generated by income connected with the company in one way or another.

From the municipal authorities' viewpoint, Minamata disease constituted a blot on both the company and the city. Every effort had to be made to rid the city of its dark, unwholesome image. The voices of the patients were to be stifled, and the very term "Minamata disease" avoided. The authorities even seriously considered trying to change the name of the disease.

The following incident epitomizes the city's callous attitude. The man in charge of general affairs at the Chisso plant called the Hygiene Department of the city office while the department head was out. Michiko's friend Akazaki answered the phone, and the Chisso representative told him that a crew from a commercial television network in Tokyo was coming to film Minamata-disease patients. He said he understood that Akazaki was to be the crew's guide and let it be known that Chisso considered the matter closed: "We don't want to dig all that up again at this late date. Don't forget," he added, "the ties between your office and our company. You understand, don't you?"

With this the Chisso representative hung up. Though nothing specific had been said, Akazaki knew that he was being told to keep the crew away from the most seriously affected patients. He later asked the members of the crew if they had informed Chisso of their plans and received a firm no. This could only mean that word had been leaked from the city office.

Though he still felt as if Michiko were leading him to the edge of an abyss full of howling demons, Akazaki felt he had to try to hinder the coverup he sensed was being attempted. He took the crew to see a bedridden victim living alone in a squalid hut in a community few outsiders visited. The TV reporter could scarcely believe his eyes. "Mr. Akazaki, this is horrible. I never expected anything like this," he exclaimed, appalled. Tense and excited, the crew began filming.

4. Witnesses to Folly

Michiko knew most of the hundred-odd patients, many of whom were destitute, and paid frequent visits to their homes. Since the authorities were trying to cover up the situation, her visits and writings elicited increasing pressure from local supporters of Chisso. Her family was plagued by nuisance telephone calls and threatening letters. Some critics told her she was stirring up unnecessary trouble and advised her to stop writing about the disease and mind her own business. Others accused her of harming her fellow citizens, since failure of the Chisso plant would hurt everyone.

These charges caused Michiko's aging parents acute suffering. When he had had a little too much to drink, her father, Kametaro, would rail at her: "You turned into a communist after you got married and started fighting with Chisso. Once upon a time you'd have been strangled in your sleep. I thought you'd make a better wife than this. You go around writing about other people's problems and don't give a damn what's happening to your own family. Are you trying to kill us?" He would end by muttering, "I'm so ashamed! What will people say?"

Michiko's mother, Haruno, always tried to calm the drunk and raging old man, saying their daughter was only doing what she felt she had to in order to relieve the suffering of others and urging him not to speak so harshly. But her efforts only caused him to turn his wrath on her. A quarrel usually ensued. But Kametaro must have known he could not change his daughter's mind. Michiko often thought he shouted at her simply to placate neighbors sympathetic to Chisso. The understanding look he sometimes gave her after a scolding led her to believe his bitter words did not reflect his true thoughts.

The Minamata-disease issue had created a whirlwind engulfing Michiko's family and upsetting the domestic routine according to which she had budgeted, prepared meals, and made clothes for everyone. Her days were so filled with information gathering and visits to patients that she had no time for household duties. Organizing the notes she had made that day and writing them up in manuscript form frequently kept her up most of the night. The numerous patients and other people involved with the problem who called at their house also imposed a burden on her mother, who had to receive them.

But it was Michiko's husband, Hiroshi, who was most cruelly buffeted by the whirlwind. Until she had become involved in the Minamata issue, apart from occasional attendance at a poetry meeting Michiko had been the model of a devoted, stay-at-home wife. Now, however, she was rarely at home even in the evening and was never there waiting for him when he returned from a day's teaching at school. In the old days she had always greeted him at the door with a word of comfort and gratitude for his hard work, cheering him and relieving his fatigue. Now he made his weary way home to find not his wife but his old mother-in-law preparing the evening meal. When Michiko had done the cooking, he had had delicious treats to nibble with his evening sakè. But no more. The slapdash meals his mother-in-law prepared were unappetizing. His son, Michio, also missed the warm, friendly dinners he used to enjoy with his mother and father.

Never having come into direct contact with the patients and therefore unaware of their suffering, Hiroshi quite naturally resented the disease for taking his wife from him. In addition, the principal and vice-principal of the school at which he taught, eager to stay on the good side of the Chisso executives whose children were pupils there, frequently made barbed comments and told him to make his wife stop writing about the disease. The local board of education also pressured him.

When some of his acquaintances callously told him they would never put up with a wife so involved with Minamata-disease patients that she neglected her husband, Hiroshi was thrown into turmoil. He resented having his family lumped together with those embroiled in ordinary domestic problems. At the same time, he wondered how long he should allow the present situation to continue.

Although he was a gentle, uncomplaining man, Hiroshi could not conceal his disappointment over his wife's estrangement from the family. Finally, unable to tolerate her total absorption in the Minamata cause, he began to drink heavily. On the few occasions that he and Michiko had a little time together, they generally quarreled. Once Hiroshi shouted, "Forget about Minamata disease! Is it so important you have to neglect your family for it?" Irritated, he tore up the manuscript Michiko was working on.

When he saw that she was adamant, Hiroshi began arguing that if she had to keep pursuing the issue, she should at least make time for her household duties as well. But Michiko replied that the problem was too important for half measures. "I just can't let it go on," she explained. "People are suffering without being given a chance to speak out. They are being killed by the poison the Chisso factory pumps out. Our gentle sea, our mother, has been ruined. I simply can't let Chisso get away with it. I can't ignore the suffering of the patients even if it means a few companies like Chisso have to shut down."

Gradually Hiroshi weakened in the face of his wife's unbending determination. He sensed a strange urgency in the way she spoke of the patients' suffering. Nonetheless, though consciously he understood the nobility of trying to alleviate their anguish, he could not help feeling dissatisfied with a wife who had no time for her own family.

Sometimes he and Michiko would argue late into the night, when everyone else in the neighborhood was fast asleep. As their talk grew more heated, he would drink himself senseless. Laying down her pen and looking tenderly at his innocent sleeping face, Michiko would think back to the beginning of their relationship. Sometimes she would sense that she had gone awry. A man had a right to criticize a wife who refused to look after her own family. Given a choice between her duties as a wife and her concern for the Minamata patients, she ought to stay at home and take care of her family. What her husband said was right in terms of conventional wisdom. When she saw things in this light, Michiko felt deeply guilty and sorry for her husband.

But having plunged into the abyss, Michiko no longer had a choice. She had to walk on with the victims. She would close her eyes and recompose herself. Possessed by their spirits, she had become the patients' chronicler. Once she took up her pen to write their silent indictment of those responsible for their anguish, she was trapped in their realm of ordeal. Not even her beloved husband could recall her from the hell through which she traveled with the spirits of the sufferers. She could not help weeping when she thought of the world of horrors into which she had been drawn and the heavy karma she bore. Looking at her sleeping husband, she would murmur, "Forgive me. I can't help myself. But I know someday you'll understand."

With Michiko away so much, Hiroshi found it hard to stay at home and took to going out drinking with Akazaki. Though Hiroshi was usually taciturn, once he had some liquor in him he would talk about his unhappiness. This topic became an unbreachable wall limiting their conversation. On one occasion Akazaki put down his drink and, looking hard at Hiroshi, said firmly, "No one would do anything to help the patients if Michiko stopped writing. She's in a very difficult position, and you should be the one to give her the most understanding. If you don't support her, nobody else will."

Hiroshi did not need Akazaki to tell him this. He knew he ought to be his wife's staunchest ally. She had put the Minamata issue before everything else and had gone too far to turn back. Hiroshi also thought that someday her enthusiasm would wane. But her great mission now was to help the patients. No one had the right to destroy the dignity of human life. Chisso was riding roughshod over the servile citizens of Minamata while concealing its actions from the outside world. Michiko was right: they could not ignore the victims' suffering. She herself was being persecuted; as her husband he should help her as much as he could. Giving her a free hand would bring her more happiness than anything else. Hiroshi even began to envy his wife for having a great, all-consuming goal. The ardor with which she strove to carry out her mission gave her a greater beauty than he had ever seen in her before. Until now he had been a selfish, demanding husband. He resolved to do his best to help her even if he had to suffer for it.

Hiroshi became an official in the teachers' union and began to play an active role in the Minamata-disease cause, visiting patients at home when her writing kept Michiko too busy. His involvement with the patients grew still deeper after he was transferred to Fukuro Middle School, located in an area where cases were especially numerous. Gradually he became a trusted confidant and did much to help the unfortunate sufferers. Although advised to take the examination for promotion to vice-principal on several occasions, he always refused because such a promotion would entail so much administrative work that he would no longer be able to help care for Minamata-disease patients.

The relationship between Hiroshi and Michiko came to resemble that between Kenzo Hashimoto and his wife, Itsue Takamure (1894–1964), a historian and feminist known for her four-volume masterpiece *Josei no Rekishi* (Women in History). Takamure, a native of Kumamoto Prefecture and one of Michiko's idols (Michiko dreamed of writing her biography), had secluded herself in what she called her "house in the forest," where she had written her history and *Hi no Kuni no Onna no Nikki* (Diary of a Woman from the Land of Fire), while her husband had sacrificed his own interests to cooperate with and serve her. After her death he lived in Minamata as custodian of his wife's literary heritage and seemed to find joy in the knowledge that he had supported her in her great work.

Hashimoto himself remarked on the similarity of the two women in their modesty and inner strength. He said that the pure flame of the Minamata movement would grow as long as there was someone like Michiko who believed firmly in human dignity and who attempted to transmit to future generations the truth about the appalling disease. He saw Michiko as a woman in the same mold as his wife, who had given herself to the feminist movement. He said that everyone like Michiko was a drop in a clear, swelling fountain of struggle in behalf of the victims of Minamata disease.

Although perhaps less self-sacrificing than Hashimoto, Hiroshi decided to do all he could to allow Michiko to devote herself to her mission without outside worries. After a family discussion, Michiko was formally released from all domestic duties. Hiroshi asked Michiko's younger sister, Taeko, who had been working in a textile plant in Gifu Prefecture, to come live with them and help out. One factor behind this decision was the condition of Michiko's mother, who had high blood pressure and could no longer manage the house and the constant stream of visitors. Taeko liked taking care of people, and with her arrival sunshine returned to the family for a time.

Things went less well for Akazaki. Unable to understand why he had to devote so much of his time to Minamata-disease patients and neglect his family, his wife left him and their daughter, who was crippled from infantile paralysis. Akazaki himself was transferred to a remote mountain branch of the city office, where, working as a radio operator, he drank himself to the brink of despair. Even while working there, however, he stayed in touch with developments in Minamata. Later, when the radio station was closed down, he returned to the city office, where he was treated as coolly as before. Nonetheless, he never abandoned the Minamata patients.

At the time that Michiko was making the rounds of patients' homes a young man named Jun Ui, having noticed Kumamoto University's announcement that organic mercury was causing a strange new illness, went to Minamata to investigate for himself. He was no stranger to the problems caused by dumping pollutants into the sea. After majoring in applied chemistry at the University of Tokyo, he had joined Nippon Zeon and been sent to work at the company's Takaoka plant, which produced vinyl chlorides. He himself had seen mercury dumped into the nearby sea without a second thought. Upon learning of the possible effects of such actions, he felt a painful sense of responsibility.

The idea that the mercury he had seen poured into the sea could cause the kind of suffering seen in Minamata filled him with profound guilt. He wanted to do something to atone for his thoughtlessness. Thus he decided to go to Minamata to make a scientific study of the situation. Resigning from Nippon Zeon, he first returned to graduate school for additional study and then, using money saved from part-time jobs, traveled to Minamata in April 1960. Akazaki arranged for him to borrow a bicycle from the city office.

When Ui visited Minamata again in 1962, he stumbled across some important information. He and a young photographer named Shisei Kuwabara, who was making a visual record of Minamata victims, called on a doctor at the Chisso hospital. While they were there Ui noticed a memorandum stamped "Staff Only" lying on the doctor's desk. It read: "Effluent from acetaldehyde plant contains 10 ppm mercury. Cats given this effluent to drink develop symptoms closely resembling those of Minamata disease."

Ui was startled. Although he knew of Kumamoto University's organic-mercury theory, this was the first he had heard of experiments performed within Chisso. Because the company had been conducting a consistent coverup ever since concluding its "condolence gift" agreement with victims in December 1959, this information had never been made public. The memorandum pertained to the data Hosokawa had discovered in his work on cat 400 in the fall of 1959. Kuwabara photographed the memorandum when the doctor was out of the room for a few minutes.

With the photograph in his possession, Ui immediately flew to Iyo, on the island of Shikoku, to talk with Hosokawa, who had returned to his hometown after leaving Chisso. The doctor examined the photo and listened, eyes closed, as Ui asked him to verify the content of the memorandum. Then he said quietly, "It's true. There's no mistake."

When he heard this, Ui was struck again by the destruction science causes when applied without humane concern. Perhaps Hosokawa read Ui's mind. The doctor told Ui that when he had realized that Chisso was unwilling to alter its policies despite his warning of the inevitable loss of life if pollution continued, he had resigned his position as the hospital's director. Before they parted, Hosokawa urged Ui to meet Michiko, describing her as "a woman totally dedicated to the Minamata-disease problem" and adding that he held her in the highest esteem.

Ui was eager to publish the important cat-experiment data, now confirmed by Hosokawa, but was uncertain how to go about it in view of the prevailing blackout on information about the disease. He also knew that any definitive evidence of Chisso's culpability would have incalculable repercussions. Then he was asked to write a commentary to a collection of Kuwabara's photographs documenting Minamata disease, which was published in 1965 by San'ichi Shobo. In his text, though nervous about the effect it might produce, he mentioned "secret experiments on cats." But in spite of the vividness with which Kuwabara's lens had captured the patients' misery, the book sold poorly and almost no one noticed Ui's brief allusion to the coverup.

Ui's most painful discovery, in the course of his efforts to trace the cause of Minamata disease, was the realization that science, which he had considered sacred, could be made the tool of money and power, as in the case of scientists who had devised false theories to help Chisso deflect public attention from the true root of the problem. He could not condone the way some men, while supposedly studying the disease, had accepted money from Chisso for overseas research. Some had even earned doctorates for research on the disease, after which they had promptly ceased to show any interest in the problem. To Ui's way of thinking, such people had bartered away both conscience and truth, perverting science from its true purpose of serving humanity.

Ui knew that if he continued his search for the truth he was bound to come into conflict with the Establishment and with other scientists. He had no illusions about the chilly reception he would receive from Tokyo University, a citadel of the Establishment, if he continued on his present course. But he decided he wanted to be able to hold his head high as a human being even if it meant never rising above the lowly rank of assistant at the university. Recalling Akazaki, who was treated as an outcast by the Minamata city office because he condemned Chisso's policy and who, at the age of fifty, had never been promoted to an administrative post, he realized that courage and a clear eye are all that are needed in the pursuit of truth.

Local journalists and Chisso technicians, as well as Hosokawa, had told Ui about a woman named Michiko Ishimure who wrote feverishly on the subject of Minamata disease. He resolved to see her, but before doing so he read her article "Strange Illness," published in *Circle Village* in 1960. Amazed, he exclaimed, "I could never have brought myself to write this!" He was astounded that a lone woman had been able to peer behind Chisso's iron curtain and boldly describe the victims' sufferings.

One day he called on Michiko. As luck would have it, she was at home, writing in the dimly lit shed she used as a study. Having believed herself almost entirely alone in her concern, she was encouraged by the fact that a young scientist had come all the way from Tokyo for the sake of a group of obscure patients in distant Minamata. Hiroshi joined them, and the three lost track of the time as they heatedly discussed Chisso, its vicious actions, and ways to help the patients. Later Michiko took Ui to the homes of some of the patients, whose condition impressed him anew with the dreadful harm mercury can do to the human body. The sight of these people suffering in abject poverty made him ashamed of the comfortable life he had enjoyed as a graduate student.

His mission as a scientist, Ui felt, was to discover why this hideous destruction of human life had been condoned. As he told Michiko, he wanted to leave a record showing that such folly could lead to the annihilation of humanity. She had her task as a writer; he must provide the scientific data to corroborate her testimony. Together, their writings must constitute both a testament to the devastation wreaked on humanity and the environment by the blind pursuit of profit and a requiem for those who had already died of Minamata disease.

Michiko and Akazaki eagerly helped Ui organize the mountain of data he had collected for his report on Minamata disease. He had a hard time finding a publisher, however, apparently because of the taboo on the subject. Finally the monthly magazine *Goka* agreed to run his report as a series beginning in 1964. Because open defiance of the Establishment and the scientists who served it was difficult at the time, Ui used the pen name Hachiro Tomita—or Tomita Hachiro, read in the customary Japanese order. With deliberate irony, he had chosen ideographs that can also be read *tonda yaro*, which means "outrageous guy." And that is what Ui proved to be, quietly restoring in proof passages the editors had deleted as controversial. His hard work paid off when a leading publisher, Sanseido, issued the articles in book form under the title *Kogai no Seijigaku: Minamata-byo o Otte* (The Politics of Pollution: Tracking Down Minamata Disease) in 1968. In his afterword, Ui acknowledges that he could never have written the book without the cooperation of such sincere and courageous fighters in the cause as Michiko Ishimure and Hajime Hosokawa.

Everyone who visited Michiko was astonished by her house. Opening the creaky front door and standing in the small dirt-floored entranceway, one could see the whole interior, from the kitchen area to the family Buddhist altar. The one-story building had no ceiling and no true room partitions. The shabbiness of the house was all the more noticeable because the dwellings around it had been rebuilt and modernized.

Although Michiko was sometimes embarrassed to receive out-of-town visitors there, the dilapidated little house was dear to her because it bore witness to her family's sufferings and hardships. It had been their home ever since they had moved to Minamata from the Amakusa Islands. Michiko was satisfied with it as it was. Furthermore, she told herself, it suited someone writ-

ing about the sufferings of the impoverished victims of Minamata disease. Sometimes she said with a smile, "The whole thing
would fall apart if a cat ran up one of the pillars." If the house
did collapse, she thought, they could always rebuild it, though
she realized very well the bitter criticism she, the chronicler of
the poor, would face if she ever erected a new house.

Michiko's study was housed in a lean-to originally used as a
tool shed. This was the birthplace of *Paradise of the Bitter Sea*. Part
of the book was first published in serial form under the title
"Umi to Sora no Aida Ni" (Between Sea and Sky) in the first
four issues of a local monthly magazine, *Kumamoto Fudoki* (November 1965 through February 1966). The journal's editor and
publisher, Kyoji Watanabe, had been introduced to Michiko's
writings by the poet Gan Tanigawa.

Watanabe described his first visit to her study as follows:

> When I first called on Michiko, in the fall of 1965, her study
> made a great impression on me. Of course it was nothing
> like a study in the usual sense. It was just a tiny wood-floored
> room tacked onto one side of the house, and a rickety book-
> shelf blocked most of the light from the window. It looked
> like the kind of retreat a young girl who loved literature might
> contrive for herself in what little space the rest of the family
> would let her use. There was barely room to sit down, and
> the poor lighting must have been ruinous to her eyes. But this
> was the only space the family could allow a housewife who
> stubbornly refused to give up literature and poetry. It was here
> that she did her writing.

"Between Sea and Sky" was based on notes Michiko made
when she and Akazaki visited Minamata-disease patients. Every
month Michiko delivered thirty or forty pages to the magazine's
office. At first Watanabe assumed her manuscript would only be
slightly reworked notes. But after reading the first installment, he
realized with excitement that he was seeing the birth of a masterpiece that was certain to have a great impact. Formerly an
editor at the *Yomiuri Shimbun* newspaper, he was familiar with

many writing styles, but Michiko's prose had a force he had never come across before.

On her first encounter with patients in Minamata Municipal Hospital in May 1959, when the sight of the fisher Tsurumatsu Kama had pierced her to the heart, she had been drawn into the world of Minamata-disease sufferers. Having visited most of the patients many times, she had come to feel their suffering as if it were her own. That is why she decided to become their chronicler, listening to them and writing what they could not. Indeed, she went further, entering into a dialogue with their souls and gazing into the abyss of their sorrow with her own eyes. The writings that eventually became *Paradise of the Bitter Sea* constitute a record of what she saw there.

To express the patients' deep anger effectively, Michiko developed a distinctive writing style that made use of the poetic spirit Tanigawa had cultivated in her. The results are apparent in the following passage from "Yuki's Testimony," which concerns Yuki Sakagami, the first patient Michiko talked to.

Ever since I got sick, I've loved my husband more than ever. I give him everything people bring me. My mouth quivers so bad I can't eat, anyway, so I give it all to him. He takes good care of me. I'm his second wife. I came from Amakusa. We hadn't been married three years before I got this strange disease. I feel terrible about it.

I can't keep my kimono closed by myself. My arms and my whole body shake like this all the time. I don't tell them to. They just do it by themselves. But he fixes my clothes for me and says, "Poor thing, it's got so you can't do anything at all. You ought to wear underpants." And then he puts them on me.

It was good out on the sea. It was really good. I'd give anything if I could be the way I used to be and work and row our boat. It breaks my heart to be the way I am now.

I can't even take care of myself when I get my period. A doctor from Kumamoto University came to look at me. I told him this disease was making me crazy. I asked him to do something to stop me from having periods. But he wouldn't do it. Said it wouldn't be good for me. I can't even wash out my sanitary belt. I'm so embarrassed about it.

If I don't work, we can't make ends meet. I have the feeling my body is slowly moving away from the rest of the world. I can't grip anything with my hands. I can't hold my husband's hand or hug my son. That's bad enough, but I can't even hold my own bowl or chopsticks. I can't put my feet on the ground and walk. I feel like I'm floating. It scares me. I feel like I'm drifting away from the world, all alone. It makes me so sad. You'll never know how sad it makes me. But I do love my husband. He's all I've got to hold onto.

I want to work. I really loved using my own arms and legs out on the water—my husband steering in the stern and me rowing. We'd go out to pull up the squid traps and octopus pots. We'd get some gray mullet, too. . . . Now, a squid's short-tempered. The minute you pull him up he's squirting that black ink at you. The octopus is a lot smarter. When you pull the pot up he hugs the bottom. He looks up at you but he won't come out. You can call him and tell him it's time, but he just stays in there. You can tap the bottom of the pot, but it won't do any good. Finally when you've had enough you pry him off the bottom with a scoop-net handle and out he comes. But then he scuttles off fast as lightning. Eight legs, and he never tangles them up! After you chase him around enough practically to swamp the boat, you finally catch him and put him in the basket. But as you row along, he comes out again and sits on the basket lid, smug as you like. I tell him, "Get back in that basket. You're in my boat now, and that means you're mine." But he just sits there looking sideways and pouting. You get to love the creatures you catch for food. It was really nice on the sea.

I get someone to put me to bed at night so I can sleep. But sometimes the blankets slip off. No one in the room can use their hands, so we can't put them back. Some people can't talk. They can't even let anybody know their blankets have slipped off. They just lie there with their eyes open. It's awful. We lie there with tears in our eyes, like fish washed up on shore. If we fall out of bed, we stay on the floor all night if the nurse is tired and has gone to sleep.

In the evenings I think about the sea more than anything. It was good being on the sea. In spring and summer all kinds of flowers bloom in the sea. Our sea is so beautiful! . . . In the summer, around our point, you can smell the shore everywhere. A lot better than the smell of some office building. At low tide you can see barnacles, and sea anemones and sea pines blooming like flowers. . . . Sea anemones look like chrysanthemums. Sea pines spread beautiful branches on the underwater cliffs. Some seaweeds look like spirea and some look like bamboo groves. The undersea world has four seasons just like the world on land. I'll bet the Dragon Palace of the fairy tales really exists on the bottom of the sea. The beautiful dream people, too. I never get tired of the sea.

Fresh water from springs in the cliffs of the small islands flows into the strong sea tides. In the early spring a seaweed called *aosa* grows on the rocks where the waters mingle. Of all the shore smells, I love best the way *aosa* smells in spring when it's drying in the sun at low tide. We'd snap the *aosa* off the rocks and pick the oysters underneath. With a little soy sauce they make a wonderful broth. City people don't know what's good till they've tasted a steaming bowl of that soup. For us, spring hadn't come till we'd practically burned our tongues on some.

I want to use my own arms and legs to go rowing out after *aosa* just one more time. I want to go so bad I could cry. Just one more time.

5. SOLIDARITY AND SCHISM

ONE DAY early in 1963 the fragrance of lily of the valley floated through the corridors of the special ward of Minamata Municipal Hospital housing Minamata-disease patients. Deeply touched by an article on the victims of this strange illness written by Michiko and published in a girls' magazine, a group of students from Hokusei Gakuen, a private girls' school in the city of Sapporo on the northern island of Hokkaido, had traveled all the way to Minamata with flowers for the patients. Earlier, the students had sent money and strings of a thousand folded-paper cranes, a traditional symbol of longevity.

The girls stood speechless before the patients. Lips tight with suppressed emotion, they handed the flowers to one of the bedridden patients. She accepted them with trembling hands, tears streaming down her face.

Among the onlookers was a primary school teacher named Fumiko Hiyoshi, who had been visiting a pupil's mother hospitalized that day. On her way out of the building she noticed a commotion and, peering into the special ward, witnessed the encounter between the Minamata-disease patients and the Hokkaido schoolgirls.

This was the first time Hiyoshi had seen Minamata-disease patients. She was shocked and saddened, especially by the sight of children condemned to a vegetablelike existence, poisoned by organic mercury absorbed through the mother's placenta before birth. Their tiny twisted bodies struck her heart with a pity rendered more poignant by the memory of the healthy children she taught every day. She left the hospital weeping.

For the next two weeks Hiyoshi slept little, tormented by visions of the suffering children. Thinking of the grief the mothers of those small victims must feel, she resolved to try to build a citizens' support movement. She decided to resign her teaching post and run for the city council in the election scheduled for April that year. Thanks to the support of local fishers and the families of Minamata-disease patients, she was elected.

Michiko advised Hiyoshi that the best way to help would be to establish a citizens' group to help the patients. Hiyoshi agreed that in view of the animosity some citizens felt toward the patients, such a group would be the only way to provide the assistance needed. The patients themselves, however, hearts hardened by years of isolation, showed little interest at first. Michiko and Akazaki understood their frustration and suspicion better than anyone else, and Hiyoshi was convinced that a viable organization could be created if these two served as a link to the patients. With Michiko's encouragement and support, Hiyoshi began diligently expounding the patients' plight on street corners and in the chambers of the city council. Gradually, despite the prevailing coolness, she caught the attention of a few sympathetic citizens.

An external factor made the creation of a citizens' group especially urgent. Word reached Minamata that representatives of patients of a second outbreak of the disease, caused by mercury contamination of the Agano River, in Niigata Prefecture, were planning to visit the city in January 1968. An organization was essential if Minamata, the first place in which the disease had occurred, was to offer the visitors a proper welcome.

On the night of January 12, 1968, Michiko and Hiyoshi called a meeting in the Minamata Municipal Education Center to establish the Citizens' Council for Minamata Disease Countermeasures. About thirty people attended, including doctors, educators, city-office employees, labor-union members, and homemakers. Representatives of the Mutual Aid Association of Families of Minamata Disease Patients, founded in 1958, were also invited. Hiyoshi was named chair. Tsutomu Matsumoto, who worked in the Construction Division of the city office and was a friend of Akazaki's, was designated secretary general.

Finally, after years of neglect, the Minamata-disease patients saw fellow citizens extending a helping hand. In a voice choked with tears, a representative of the Mutual Aid Association said, "If only this organization had existed ten years ago, all our suffering would have . . . it's too late now." Everyone in the audience looked down in silence.

In a leaflet distributed to all the patients' homes, Michiko wrote on behalf of the Citizens' Council: "As citizens of Minamata, we are deeply ashamed that in the fourteen years since the initial outbreak none of us have done anything to relieve the suffering of those stricken."

Through the tireless efforts of Hiyoshi and Matsumoto, the organization gradually expanded. They were at the hub of a four-team operation: a study team responsible for preparing for the trial occasioned by a suit filed against Chisso in June 1969 by twenty-nine families, a team responsible for patient care and aid, and public-relations and financial-affairs teams.

At first the council members tended to see the patients not as suffering families or individuals but as the collective symbol of Minamata disease itself. Perhaps this was inevitable, since the members' initial contacts with the patients were through formal meetings and lectures. The council members still had no real understanding of the depth of the patients' personal and family suffering. To the closemouthed patients, wary of all outsiders after having been shunned for so long, assistance offered on the basis of such flawed comprehension seemed overeager and somehow suspect. But Michiko, who had known the patients for a decade, understood them and conveyed their true needs and desires to the council members, thus enabling the members to enter more fully into the minds of those they were trying to help.

At the conclusion of one council meeting, the mother of a patient said, "I'm just beginning to understand how much you really want to help. Our hearts have been closed for a long time, and it may take just as long to open them up again. Please be patient with us." This broke the ice; suddenly animated conversation filled the air, patients and council members relating for the first time on a human level.

Although the Citizens' Council moved haltingly at first, to Michiko, who had been carrying on the struggle virtually alone for years, this widening of the circle of support seemed a tremendous reinforcement. But with a staff limited to local people, the organization had its hands full dealing with the problems presented by the growing number of patients in Minamata itself, to which its services were necessarily confined. While its daily work was important and demanded close attention, the council was not strong enough to stand up to Chisso, with its immense financial resources. Michiko realized that it was also necessary to create a larger organization to fight Chisso and carry on nationwide public-relations and fund-raising campaigns to gain support for the patients.

Kyoji Watanabe, who had edited and published *Kumamoto Fudoki* during its brief life from November 1965 to December 1966, understood Michiko's thinking. Until reading her manuscripts for "Between Sea and Sky," he had known nothing of Minamata disease. Each time he read her descriptions of the patients' plight, however, he was plunged deeper into their world. People who have suffered greatly acquire an aura of sanctity and a kind of absolute authority. To Watanabe the Minamata-disease patients' living hell as Michiko described it became a kind of sacred realm into which he felt himself being drawn.

He felt that Michiko was doing much more than simply chronicling the patients' situation and environmental pollution; she was, in effect, challenging unbridled capitalism. Michiko herself, however, was not concerned with the larger social questions that might be stirred up by exposure of the wickedness of the company responsible for the pollution and the ineptness of the government's response to the problem. She was simply driven to write by the horrors she witnessed. But the purity of her vision and the urgency of her words ripped the makeshift bandage from a gaping wound.

Watanabe was convinced that Michiko's work would blaze

the way for a new struggle to help the patients. She was gratified when he told her frankly of his compulsion to do something for them and added that, with a trial in the offing, it was crucial to publicize the patients' situation as widely as possible and create a nationwide support network.

In April 1969 Watanabe gathered twenty sympathizers at the Social Welfare Center in Kumamoto City, the prefectural capital, to set up the Association to Indict [Those Responsible for] Minamata Disease. Keikichi Honda, a teacher at the Kumamoto First High School and a close friend of Watanabe's, was chosen to be the group's official representative. Watanabe read aloud a declaration he had prepared:

> We have formed this association to take all possible measures to combat Minamata disease, which we regard as violence perpetrated against people as close to us as our own families. Accepting it as our own problem, we are resolved to give our full support to the Minamata trial. In addition to the trial campaign, we are determined to carry out all activities necessitated by the issue. We are not professional agitators or political partisans. We invite all who are concerned over Minamata disease and are seeking ways to take action to join the struggle.

This humble yet powerful message inspired those assembled to pledge their unconditional support. In response to Michiko's concern that people be informed of the patients' actual circumstances, Watanabe proposed that the group publish a periodical titled *Kokuhatsu* (Indictment), to be edited at Honda's home in Kumamoto City and distributed nationwide. It would carry all the news pertaining to Minamata disease. Watanabe himself would serve as editorial adviser, and friends on the *Kumamoto Nichinichi Shimbun*, a local daily, and the *Kyushu Daigaku Shimbun*, the Kyushu University newspaper, would write and edit articles. The periodical would be published on the twenty-fifth of each month.

Ordinarily, seven thousand copies of *Kokuhatsu* were printed, though an occasional issue ran to eighteen thousand copies. It was delivered free of charge to the homes of all patients. Printing and other costs were covered by contributions from all over Japan.

The lead article in the first issue, which appeared on June 25, 1969, was headlined "War Declared on Chisso" and reported the suit filed against Chisso in the Kumamoto District Court on June 14. This issue also carried an article by Michiko on the long years of hardship and suffering between the outbreak of the disease and the decision to take the matter to court. In almost every issue, Akazaki chronicled the experiences of patients and their families in a series of articles titled "Fukaki Fuchi yori Sakebu" (Cries from the Abyss).

Thanks to Michiko's insistence that its editorial policy center on the patients themselves, *Kokuhatsu* became a vital weapon in their struggle. With each issue, the periodical's detailed coverage of the Minamata problem captured increasing attention, and reporters from mainstream newspapers began using the publication as a news source. Fortunately, Michiko's *Paradise of the Bitter Sea*, published in January that year, had captured nationwide attention, and contributions accompanied by letters of protest against the pollution behind the disease began pouring in.

Honda, who had been drawn into the movement by Michiko's writings, published in *Kokuhatsu* the following explanation of his decision to serve as a volunteer:

I first encountered victims of Minamata disease in the initial installment of Michiko Ishimure's "Between Sea and Sky," published in the inaugural issue of *Kumamoto Fudoki* in the fall of 1965. There I was introduced to a young boy named Kyuhei Yamanaka. Over the following months I came to know an old man named Sensuke Namiki, a married couple named Yuki and Mohei Sakagami, another boy named Mokutaro Ezu, his grandmother and grandfather, and other patients and their families. The world I discovered through her writing was exactly like that of my own grandparents.

I had the greatest respect and affection for my maternal grandfather, who died in 1952 at the age of eighty-two. He was

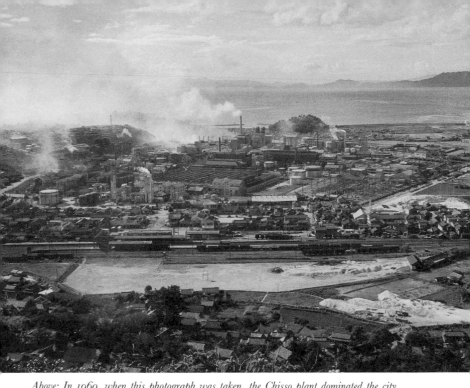

Above: In 1960, when this photograph was taken, the Chisso plant dominated the city of Minamata. In the background lie the Shiranui Sea and the Amakusa Islands. Below: The fishing hamlet of Modo, also photographed in 1960, was among the communities most heavily hit by Minamata disease. (Photos by Shisei Kuwabara)

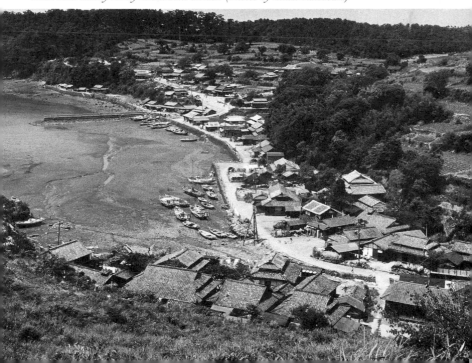

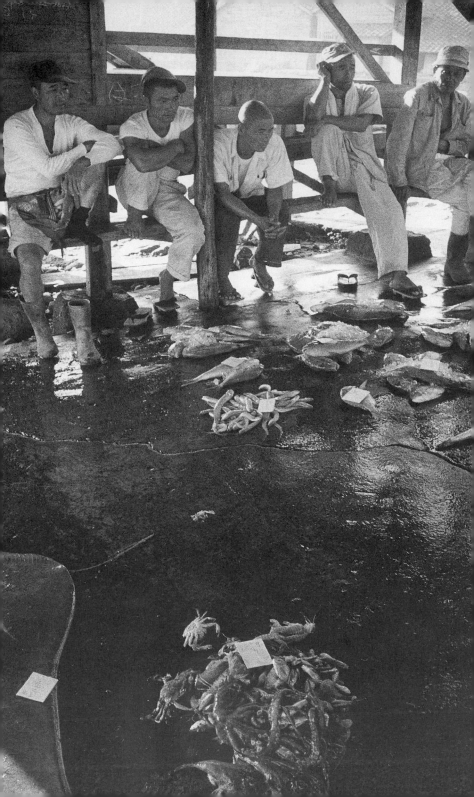

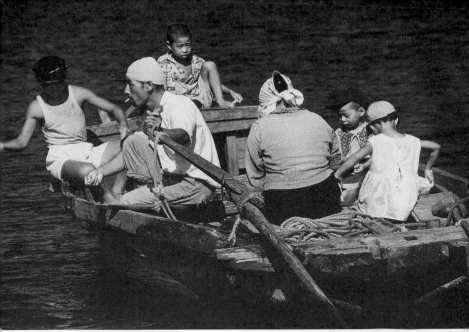

Opposite: This 1960 photograph shows glum Minamata fishers waiting to auction their meager catches from the polluted waters of the Shiranui Sea. Above: Even in 1970, when this photograph was taken, many families continued to fish in the mercury-contaminated ocean to eke out a living. Right: This careworn woman mending a fishing net was photographed in 1970. (Photos by Shisei Kuwabara)

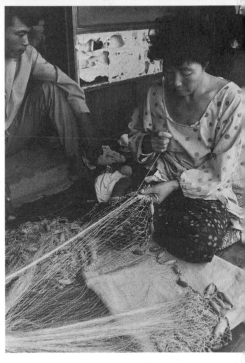

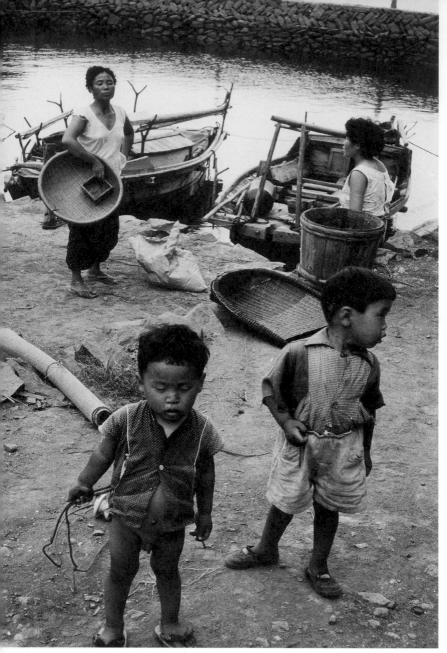

This 1960 scene of women and children in the fishing hamlet of Tsukinoura evokes the bleak poverty of such communities. (Photo by Shisei Kuwabara)

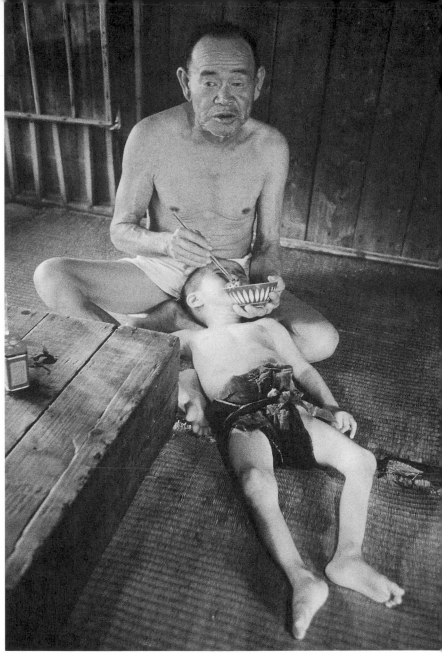

Mokutaro Ezuno, born with Minamata disease, and his grandfather were photographed at home in 1960. (Photo by Shisei Kuwabara)

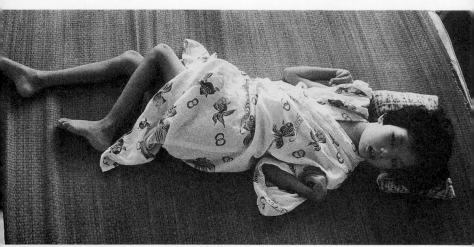

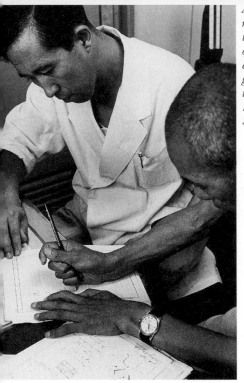

Above: Kumiko Matsunaga was afflicted with Minamata disease as a small child. This photograph was taken in 1960; she died in 1974. Left: The numbness of the fingers typical of Minamata disease makes it difficult for patients to write, as seen in this 1970 photograph. Opposite: The fisher Tsurumatsu Kama, one of the first patients Michiko Ishimure encountered, died in 1960, the year this photograph was taken. (Photos by Shisei Kuwabara)

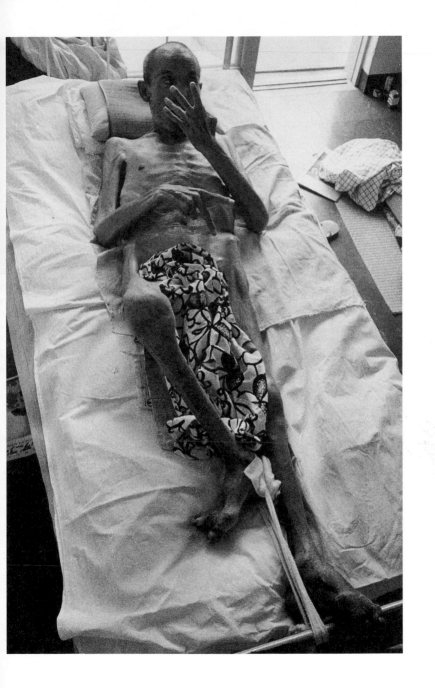

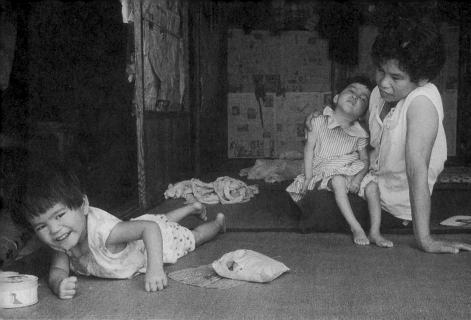

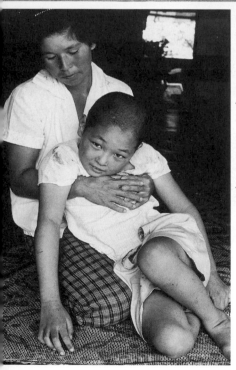

Above: Both these sisters were congenital victims of Minamata disease. The older girl (right), born in 1956, died in 1962, two years after this photograph was taken. Her sister was eventually institutionalized. Left: This boy, born in 1959 and photographed in 1970, was also congenitally afflicted. Opposite: Tomoko Kamimura, born with the disease in 1956, is pictured above with her parents and a healthy sister in 1960 and below with family and friends on January 15, 1977. (January 15 is Coming of Age Day, when young women who have turned twenty customarily don festive kimono.) She died in December 1978. (Photos by Shisei Kuwabara)

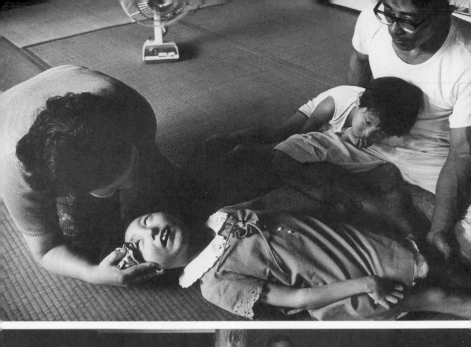

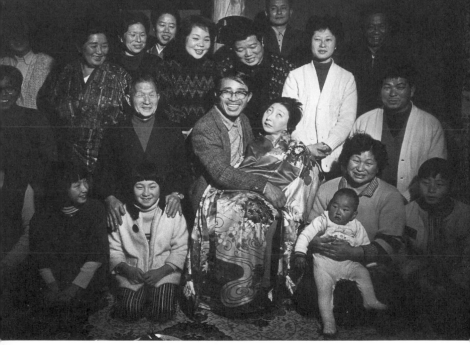

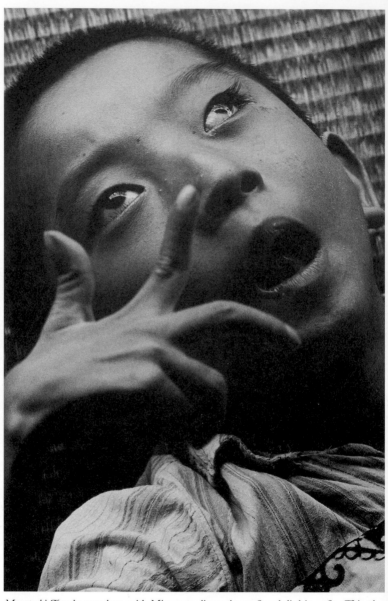

Masatoshi Tanaka was born with Minamata disease in 1956 and died in 1969. This photograph was taken in 1966. (Photo by Shisei Kuwabara)

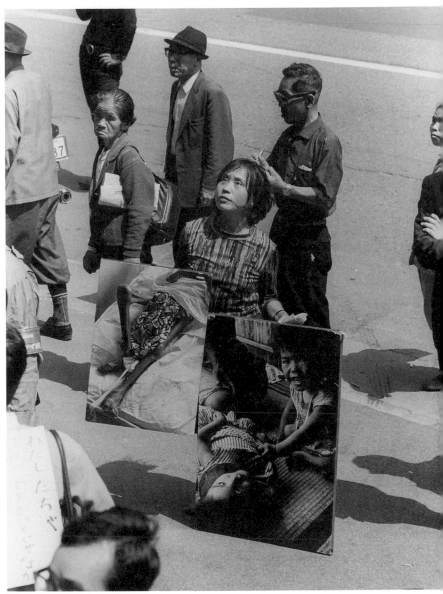

Michiko Ishimure took part in the protest in front of the Ministry of Health and Welfare on May 25, 1970. (Photo by Takeshi Shiota)

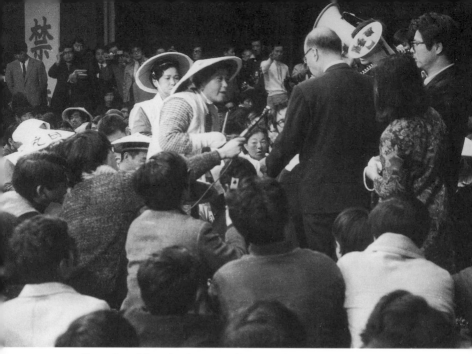

Above: One of the patients' representatives at the Chisso annual shareholders' meeting on November 28, 1970, dressed in pilgrim garb and clutching a memorial tablet, berated Chisso's president. *Below:* Black banners bearing the ideograph on *(rancor)* were raised outside Chisso's Minamata plant in November 1971. *(Photos by Takeshi Shiota)*

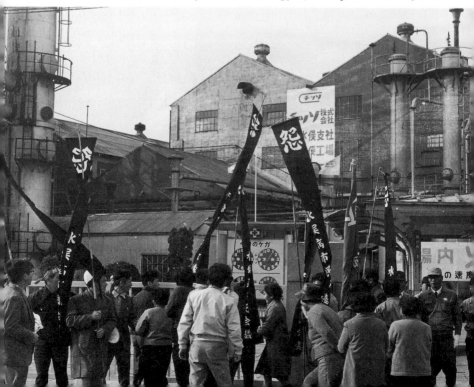

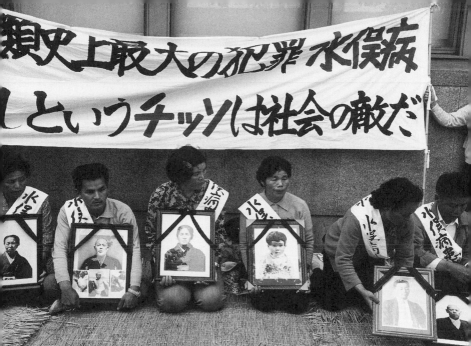

Above: Demonstrators, displaying photographs of deceased loved ones, began a sit-in at Chisso's Tokyo headquarters in December 1971. (Photo by Shisei Kuwabara) Below: Teruo Kawamoto (second from right) and other activists launched a sit-in in front of Chisso's Minamata plant in November 1971. (Photo by Takeshi Shiota)

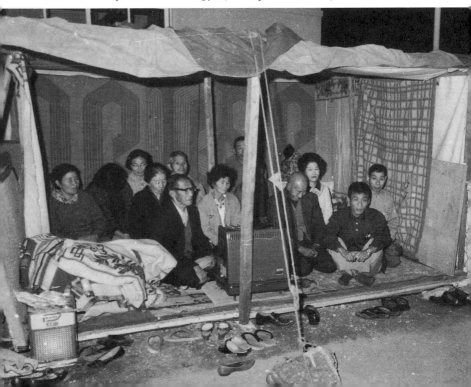

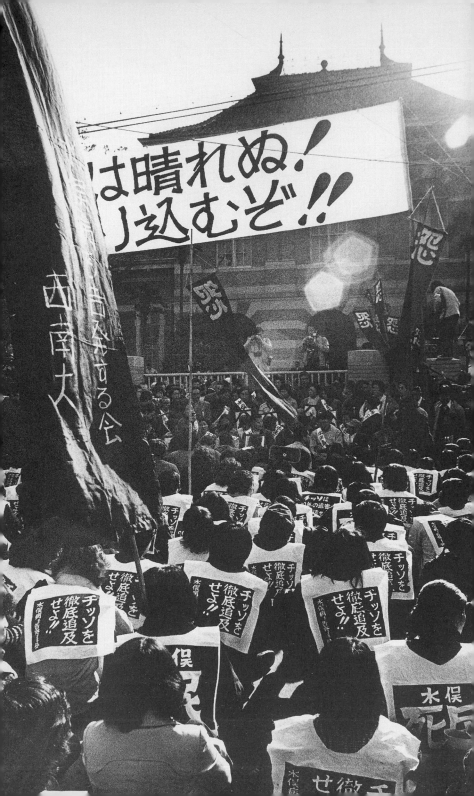

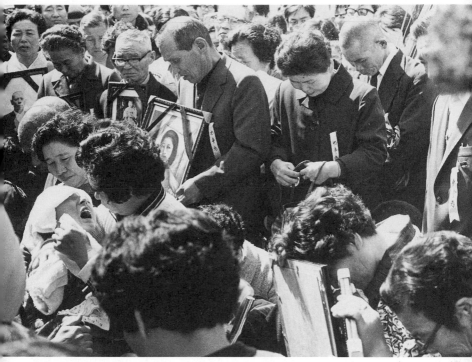

Opposite: Patients and supporters, some bearing on banners, gathered outside the Ku-mamoto District Court on March 20, 1973, the day of the verdict in the patients' suit against Chisso. Above: Despite the plaintiffs' victory, there was no rejoicing. The sor-rowful faces of those holding photographs of loved ones lost to Minamata disease testify to the toll taken by the long battle with the Establishment. In the foreground a girl born with the disease cries out in her mother's arms. (Photos by Takeshi Shiota)

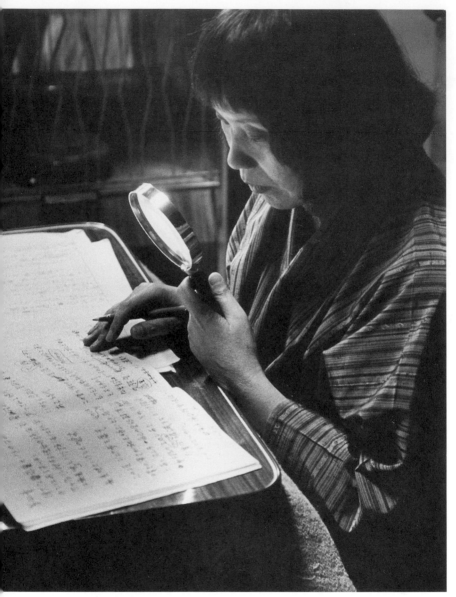

Michiko Ishimure's eyesight deteriorated until in 1976, when this photograph was taken, she could read only with the aid of a magnifying glass. (Photo by Takeshi Shiota)

an outstanding farmer who worked in the fields until the end. I felt a strong link between him and old Sensuke, whom I read about in *Kumamoto Fudoki*. Indeed, Michiko Ishimure's writings led me to feel as if Minamata disease were attacking my own grandparents' world. Though some of its customs were different, my grandparents' world was basically the same as my parents' and therefore my own world. I identified strongly with the boy Kyuhei.

I visited Tsukinoura and Yudo in Minamata for the first time in April this year. Gazing at the beautiful sea and thinking of the people who had watched the sun rise from and descend quietly into it every day for years, I asked myself how anyone could possibly forgive the needless poisoning of those waters.

The enemy is before our eyes. . . . This brazen enemy, having confirmed through secret experiments that it was indeed poisoning the sea, concealed the results and continued its actions, even issuing threatening public statements suggesting that the local people had better not jeopardize themselves by incurring its wrath. Its attitude represents the worst kind of tyrannical capitalist oppression and exploitation of the masses: the dumping of poison into local waters has exploited lives.

Wiping the blood from its lips, the oppressor and exploiter stands before us. Are we prepared to follow old custom and allow the matter to go no further than merely thinking and talking about it?

Those who refuse to fight the enemy that is before their very eyes become sheep, slavishly subservient to the Establishment. The time for thinking and talking has passed. The time for mere self-righteous verbal criticism of the Establishment is over.

I am determined to join the battle line drawn by the Citizens' Council for Minamata Disease Countermeasures. I do not know how well I can fight. But whatever I can do is bound to have an effect on my work as a teacher and to prove that I am truly alive.

Behind Michiko's desire to keep the struggle apolitical was the bitter memory of her own brush with party politics. In the naive belief that the Japan Communist Party was full of people like the poet Gan Tanigawa, she had joined the party in 1959, the year in which she had become involved in the Minamata issue. But owing to his zeal to reform the party, whose increasing bureaucracy deeply concerned him, Tanigawa was declared an antiparty element and expelled in 1960. Michiko, who wrote for Tanigawa's journal *Circle Village*, was branded an enemy of the people and left the party the same year.

The literary circle Tanigawa founded in Minamata in the mid-1950s, before Minamata disease became a social issue, ignited a strong flame of self-awareness that spread first to Michiko, then to her husband, and from them to Akazaki, his colleague Matsumoto, Chisso labor-union leader Tatsuaki Okamoto, and ultimately the entire first phase of the movement in behalf of Minamata-disease patients.

Tanigawa left Minamata in 1958, before the extent of the disease was known, and went to Chikuho, in Fukuoka Prefecture, where the coal miners' union was in danger of being destroyed. He also took part in the labor disputes at the Miike coal mine of Mitsui Mining, near Omuta, Kumamoto Prefecture. Forming a study group with Hidenobu Ueno, Kazue Morisaki, and other local writers, he founded *Circle Village* as a medium for exchange among like-minded people. Through the ideal of the "new village," he helped guide the miners' union and took part in the movement opposing reduction of the mining labor force in the name of "rationalization." During the violent struggle involving the Taisho coal miners' union, he formed the Taisho Action Group, reorganizing the union's antiauthority camp, which had been on the verge of collapse.

Tanigawa's ultimate goal was to upgrade what had been merely a cultural movement into a class-based creative movement, as he explained in an article in the first issue of *Circle Village,* published in October 1958:

We proclaim our intention of creating a village—a vast and

strange village stretching from the bonito boats of Kagoshima Prefecture [on southern Kyushu] to the firewood tow-
ers of Yamaguchi Prefecture [on southwestern Honshu]. The
cultural-creation movement in Japan is now facing a sharp
turning point. To reverse the trend toward purge and disso-
lution that has continued for the past two or three years, we
must destroy the idea that culture is ultimately the creation
of individuals and thus prepare the way for the emergence of
new groups.

The new creative unit must be the circle. Searching for
the origins of the circle in popular tradition, we discover it
in the solidarity uniting people in the lower echelons of the
community and in their organizations. . . . At present the
fragments of the old community, shattered by capitalism, are
melding into the community of the future. The circle is a
bridge. It is also the crucible in which the melding process
can take place. . . .

In the belief that the rhythms of creativity and of daily life
(labor) must harmonize, we must struggle to fill not only the
products of creative work but also the entire creative process
with the breath of the group. Ultimately, our movement must
always return to the group. Groups that return to the individual cannot be regarded as circles. The sole aim of our movement is to organize the world of creative activity.

Tanigawa approached Communist Party cultural activists with
the hope of expanding the Circle Village movement nationwide
by founding a journal that would serve as a national cultural fo-
rum, but was viciously attacked for "antiparty thought." Nonetheless, he persevered in his efforts to reorganize people and
oppose the highhanded policies of the central party authorities.
In July 1960 all the major members of the Circle Village group
were dismissed as Trotskyites and notified that their names had
been struck from the roll of the party's district committee. The
leaflet announcing this decision denounced them as enemies of
the people and accused them of having degenerated into "an
anticommunist 'left wing' provocateur group."

The Circle Village group replied by distributing a leaflet announcing the group's split from "the soulless Communist Party":

Why are people who have always believed themselves enthusiastic party members now damned as enemies of the people? Why must we exchange bitter words with our comrades in arms, with whom we have shared both sorrow and joy for so long? This has happened because the Communist Party has lost its soul. It has lost the stern, throbbing soul of individuals striving to rebuild the world from its foundations. . . . The Communist Party has consistently called the mainstream of Zengakuren [National Federation of Student Self-government Associations], now engaged in the anti–security treaty movement and the Miike coal mine dispute, a lackey of American imperialism and a provocateur intentionally sowing disorder to destroy the [party] struggle.

The party denounced as a class betrayal the campaign to raise funds for those injured when protesting Prime Minister [Nobusuke] Kishi's departure for the United States on January 16 this year to sign the revised security treaty and refused to send representatives to the funeral of Michiko Kamba, who was killed in a demonstration in front of the National Diet Building on June 15. To critics of this refusal, the party replied that sending a representative would have been tantamount to exploiting sympathy for the dead to glorify destructive activities. . . .

Attitudes toward victims of the class struggle are the most reliable measure of the conscience of individual and organization alike. Sohyo [General Council of Trade Unions of Japan] has verified that the violence perpetrated against Zengakuren members by the police at Miike on July 22 was not instigated by Zengakuren. Moreover, all the journalists on the scene protested to the police. Only the Communist Party, not surprisingly, is calling the action "Trotskyite provocation."

The party's district committee has adopted the same attitude toward the struggle against labor-force reduction in the name of rationalization at the Taisho coal mine. . . . Far from repenting its mistaken guidance, it accuses us of deviating from the party line and of defying the will of party organs. In its view, we have broken the rules and are antiparty elements because we have not done as ordered. Does the committee wish to make orders from party superiors as binding as commands handed down from the emperor? What a petty bureaucratic attitude!

To preserve the soul of the communist within us, after an arduous struggle we find ourselves compelled to come to a parting of the ways. To our bitter disappointment, the party leadership has become mired in bureaucracy.

Prevention of suffering among the working masses demands a locomotive moving ahead at full steam. We do not consider ourselves to be that locomotive, but we do believe we can be one of its parts or a piece of the coal used to fuel it. Hand in hand with comrades around the nation, we are setting out on the long road toward the creation of a truly avant-garde party.

Michiko was labeled an enemy of the people by the party's district committee for publishing "Strange Illness," her first article on Minamata disease, in *Circle Village*. Condemnation of her efforts to reveal the tragedy of the downtrodden by the very party that was supposed to represent the masses disillusioned her. As the attacks on *Circle Village* grew more virulent, the party instructed Michiko to stop submitting manuscripts to the journal and to present for party approval all manuscripts she intended to publish elsewhere. Unable to tolerate this interference with her creative freedom, Michiko left the party. She wrote the following bitter "declaration of independence":

Because Gan Tanigawa was away . . . , the Japan Communist Party's attacks on *Circle Village* in Minamata were directed mainly at me. I was even disparaged as "a mere woman." For belonging to the Circle Village group, which was openly critical of the party, and for contributing manuscripts to the [group's] journal for the benefit of the well-intentioned masses, I was accused of Trotskyite deviation and of aiding and abetting the enemy by confusing the masses. The conflict between the party's district committee and me over Tanigawa's article "Norikoerareta Zen'ei" [Beyond the Avant-garde] was both comic and tragic, as shown by the following criticism of me by a local party leader:

"The idea that one who is a member of an avant-garde party can transcend the avant-garde is tantamount to putting the Circle Village group on a level with or above the party. That is revisionist thinking. Most writers are egoists and have an inflated opinion of themselves. Which do you choose, the party or the Circle Village group, a Trotskyite organization? You should remain in the party and engage in self-criticism.

"You refuse to recognize the decision of communist parties the world over that Soviet and Chinese nuclear experiments are preferable to those conducted by American imperialists, believing that you alone are correct. Criticizing the local party authorities and defying the communist parties of the world, you assert the correctness of Gan Tanigawa's political and literary thought. You must consider yourself very grand. Through its official organs and its current drive to double membership, the party is giving its all to the attempt to succor the masses. We should like to hear the scheme with which you intend to achieve that end, working on your own outside the party."

Never having publicly declared my party affiliation, I did not bother to report this ludicrous incident to the editorial staff of *Circle Village*. A few months later, humiliated and feeling like a stray dog, I left the party.

In 1959, following Michiko's example, Hiroshi had also joined the party. But he too resigned in 1960, enraged at its public denunciation of Michiko as an enemy of the people despite her heroic efforts to help the Minamata-disease patients.

The expulsion of Tanigawa, who had organized the party's Minamata cell, followed by the resignations of Michiko and Hiroshi, dealt the party a severe blow. The Minamata cell soon broke away from the party. Having lost local support and per-

haps preoccupied with the more conspicuous security-treaty issue, the Communist Party failed to turn its attention to the appalling human suffering that tyrannical capitalism was causing
in the small city of Minamata.

Michiko and the others carried on their lonely battle with
still greater fervor. Ironically, the very purity of their struggle
may have resulted both from the Communist Party's failure to
play a vigorous role in the early phase of the movement and
from Michiko's isolation, which enabled her to define her task
in terms of the true needs of the patients. Still more ironically,
it was Tanigawa, now driven out of the party, who had first ignited the flame of the movement and spread it.

Frustrated with the revolution, Tanigawa abandoned all political activities and stopped writing. But though Michiko too
was frustrated over the difficulty of bringing about revolutionary
change, she continued to write about the sufferings of disadvan-
taged people in the lowest stratum of society. And as her repu-
tation as a writer grew, the very party that had once called her
an enemy of the people began to court her. The newspaper *Aka-
hata* (Red Flag), the oldest and most important organ of the Japan Communist Party, requested her to write for it, but she
refused, repelled by the party's twisted logic that even nuclear
weapons are justified if they are in the hands of one's allies.

6. Challenges to
the Establishment

THE KUMAMOTO prefectural government's Minamata Disease Patients Screening Board, formed in December 1959 (renamed the Pollution Victims Certification Board in 1969), which determined whether individuals were actually suffering from Minamata disease, was under Chisso's thumb and thus naturally tried to minimize the number of new cases certified, since any increase meant that Chisso would have to pay additional compensation.

By means of the "condolence gift" agreement that patients had been forced to sign in December 1959, Chisso hoped to create the impression that Minamata disease was no longer a problem. The desire to foster this notion is clearly reflected in a report issued in the mid-1960s by Haruhiko Tokuomi, a member of the Screening Board who was a professor at the Kumamoto University School of Medicine at the time. Despite the steady stream of new cases, Tokuomi wrote: "Since no new cases of Minamata disease have been seen since 1961, the outbreak appears to have ended."

In December 1959 Chisso had installed purification equipment designed to give the impression that no more mercury was being dumped into the sea; thus the Screening Board probably felt bound to follow Chisso's line by denying the emergence of new cases. The minutes of one meeting include a statement of agree-

ment that, since compensation was involved, the "utmost cau-
tion" was necessary in certifying new patients. Clearly, the board
was supporting Chisso's attempt to put the Minamata-disease
affair behind it.

Akazaki learned how greatly the Screening Board was influenced by Chisso when, arriving at work at the city office one
morning in 1964, he overheard the chief clerk of the General
Affairs Division say, in a hung-over voice, "The board meeting
last night was quite something. Those Chisso people really know
how to do things! After the meeting they took us to the best
cabaret in Kumamoto City."

Akazaki could hardly believe his ears. He knew a board meeting had been held in an expensive Japanese-style restaurant in
Kumamoto City the previous evening. Those present had included the head of the prefectural government's Hygiene Department, the director of the Minamata public health office, the
director of Minamata Municipal Hospital, Professor Tokuomi,
and—significantly—the director of the Chisso hospital.

Decisions to certify patients, which had to be unanimous, were
made on the basis of the individual patient's application and a
diagnostic report from Minamata Municipal Hospital. After a
perfunctory discussion, certification of all new applicants was de-
ferred. Then a Chisso employee had the food and drink brought
in. The ensuing party was marked by a mood of general satisfaction that no new cases had been certified. Later the board
members, by then quite tipsy, staggered on to a cabaret.

The city office was in charge of the budget for Minamata-
disease patients but certainly did not have the resources to pay
for parties on this scale. Akazaki realized all too well what the
chief clerk had meant when he said, "Those Chisso people really know how to do things!"

Many of those afflicted with Minamata disease preferred enduring their lot to applying for certification, a step that left them
open to the opprobrium and discrimination suffered by patients.
When they found themselves unable to pay for further treatment and applied in desperation, they were likely to be accused
of greed. The voluntary-application system, instituted in 1960,

was thus an effective way of minimizing the number of certifications.

Furthermore, the Minamata Municipal Hospital diagnostic reports submitted with the applications were generally inscribed "No details known" or specified such conditions as encephalitis, cerebral palsy, or "senility." In one case, a woman whose child was obviously seriously affected by mercury poisoning filed an application, but because her child's condition had been diagnosed as encephalitis the application was ignored for ten years.

Patients whose applications were turned down received nothing but a postcard stamped "Rejected." The number of rejected patients grew. Many so-called latent patients who suffered in silence, afraid to submit applications, also lived along the shores of the Shiranui Sea. Estimating their total was impossible.

A man named Teruo Kawamoto, whose father had died an uncertified victim of Minamata disease, finally decided to challenge the Establishment. In 1965 he appealed to the Minamata public health office and the city office for posthumous recognition of his father's status as a patient, but the Screening Board refused to consider the case. Even when indications of Minamata disease were discovered in autopsies, no further investigation was made. Such cases were considered closed.

Unable to countenance this disregard of human rights, Kawamoto appealed in vain to the district human rights commission in 1968 and to the prefectural commission in 1969. He also mailed questionnaires to members of the Screening Board asking them to explain their reasons for refusing to deal with the cases of deceased patients. The only reply he received was that board members could not respond to individual requests for information regarding Minamata disease.

Kawamoto himself suffered from the disease. Since 1956 he had been troubled by tremors and numbness of his hands and feet. Anger at the Screening Board's refusal to investigate deceased victims led him to apply for certification in 1968, but he met with a chilly reception from the panel of doctors who examined him. They asked why he had waited so long to apply. His explanation that outside pressures had constrained him elicited no sympathy from these men, who seemed to think he just wanted the money he would receive as a certified patient. They suggested he was not ill at all, noting disparagingly, "But you aren't suffering any muscular spasms right now."

Kawamoto fully understood what other patients meant when they complained that gaining certification was as hard as passing the notoriously difficult entrance examination to Tokyo University. Indeed, the panel refused to consider for certification any patient who did not manifest the full range of symptoms associated with mercury poisoning—the so-called Hunter-Russell syndrome, including constriction of the field of vision, ataxia, sensory disturbances, and hardness of hearing. Kawamoto became acutely aware that the Screening Board, which should have been on the patients' side, was nothing but a tool of the Establishment.

Around this time, he read some of Michiko's writings. Encouraged by her profound compassion for those who, like him, were despised and discriminated against, he resolved to help his fellow sufferers find a way out of the darkness of neglect. Walking the sorrowful path that Michiko and Akazaki had followed earlier, Kawamoto went from house to house among the fishing hamlets to seek out victims suffering in silence. Often forgetting to eat or sleep, he devoted himself to persuading as many fellow patients as possible to apply for certification. At first he met with suspicion, as well as skepticism that anything could be done to reverse decisions already handed down from on high. Each time, he explained that he himself had applied and been turned down but that he had no intention of letting matters rest there. To give up, he said, would be tantamount to condoning Chisso, which had crippled them, robbed them of their loved ones, and polluted their beautiful sea.

Kawamoto's fervent pleas had an effect. He was able to persuade more than two dozen people to apply for certification with him, including nineteen who had never applied before. The group included seven women whose children suffered from severe congenital Minamata disease. Unfortunately, many members of the group were unable to withstand the accusations of greed leveled at them by outsiders and eventually withdrew their applications.

In the end, only eleven of the original twenty-eight remained. Kawamoto submitted their applications to the public health office on January 20, 1970. The next day, a police officer called on him and pressed him to divulge the names of the other applicants. Realizing that anyone who defied Chisso was liable to police surveillance, he felt keenly the oppressive weight of big business.

In June 1970 all the applications were turned down, but Kawamoto refused to admit defeat. He concentrated on searching for some way to censure the board for its lack of medical ethics and to invalidate its rejection of the eleven applications. Suddenly he saw a glimmer of hope. He learned that on the basis of the Administrative Appeals Law he could appeal directly to the minister of health and welfare to investigate an administrative decision. Gaining the agreement of eight of those whose applications had been rejected, he filed an official request that their complaint be investigated. With Michiko's help he began drafting a written rebuttal of the board's findings.

About a year later, Kawamoto's diligence paid off. On August 7, 1971, the newly established Environment Agency revoked the governor of Kumamoto Prefecture's rejection of these patients' applications. The agency ruled as follows:

1. The Kumamoto Prefecture Pollution Victims Certification Board misunderstands the medical concept of Minamata disease. Measures taken by the prefectural governor on the basis of that misunderstanding are legally void.

2. Overemphasizing the relationship between certification and indemnity, the board and the governor have applied the law inappropriately, and the measures the governor has taken on the basis of such application are legally void.

3. The parties requesting investigation do in fact suffer from Minamata disease.

For these three reasons, the measures taken by the governor are to be revoked and certification is to be granted.

The implication of this statement was that applicants were to be given the benefit of the doubt and that help would be forthcoming for those patients who had not yet been certified. At last the door had opened a crack.

Reflecting on Kawamoto's long efforts to move the bureaucracy, Michiko realized that those who persevere prevail in the end. Why, though, should pollution victims, whose needs would be immediately met in a nation where public welfare was truly a major concern, be compelled to wage such a long and arduous struggle? She foresaw further obstacles, since the board too had been thoroughly polluted by Chisso.

Branded a law breaker by the Environment Agency and widely viewed with suspicion, the board certified Kawamoto and his fellow complainants in October 1971. But its basic nature as a tool of the Establishment suggested that patients applying for certification in the future would still face many barriers.

On September 26, 1968, the Ministry of Health and Welfare finally issued a clear-cut statement that Chisso was responsible for Minamata disease. This cast a pall over Chisso's sympathizers, and Minamata citizens were tense with anxiety over the future of both Chisso and the city.

Two weeks before the official government opinion was issued, the city had sponsored a memorial service for victims of the disease. On the very day of the service Chisso President Yutaka Egashira, in anticipation of the government's declaration, hinted that the company might relocate its Minamata plant. This veiled threat shocked the local citizens and so heightened their animosity toward the patients that no outsiders attended the service.

On the day following the government announcement, however, Egashira unexpectedly visited the homes of some certified patients to apologize on behalf of the company—an apparent about-face after years of adamantly refusing to issue any kind of apology. He even said he was willing to discuss the subject of compensation with patients' families. Chisso's subsequent actions belied these conciliatory words, however.

Negotiations between Chisso and the Mutual Aid Association began while emotions were still running high in the city. But Chisso allowed months to pass without replying to the association's demand for payment of ¥13 million for each death and an annuity of ¥600,000 for each living patient. A plan to set up a mediating body centered on the governor of Kumamoto Prefecture fell flat when the governor, Kosaku Teramoto, refused to have anything to do with it. As the outcry against the patients' demands grew louder among local citizens, the outlook for the future of negotiations grew bleaker. By the beginning of 1969 the patients found themselves hard pressed both materially and psychologically.

Observing the situation, Michiko wondered uneasily whether the bitterness and remorse associated with the humiliating "condolence gift" agreement of 1959 would be repeated. Indeed, a plan that would have caused her great anxiety, had she known of it, was evolving. In late February 1969 the Health and Welfare Ministry announced its intention of setting up an impartial mediation committee and asked the Mutual Aid Association to sign a document promising to leave selection of the committee members entirely to the ministry and to abide by the committee's decisions. In effect, the ministry was saying that it would not mediate unless the patients agreed to this condition—which would give the ministry carte blanche and deprive the patients of the right to make any complaints whatsoever.

Within the Mutual Aid Association, reaction to this demand was mixed. Some members flatly refused to sign the document and resolved to fight to the finish against Chisso. Others felt it would be wisest to leave the matter in the ministry's hands.

That the document in question was based on a draft prepared by Chisso became clear when a Socialist member of the Diet pressed the matter. The following exchange between Noboru Agune of the Socialist Party of Japan and Kiichiro Muto, director of the Health and Welfare Ministry's Pollution Department, took place in the Committee on Social and Labor Affairs of the House of Councillors, the Diet's upper house, on March 18, 1969.

MUTO: What I handed Mr. Yamada, head of the Hygiene Department of Minamata City, Mr. Fujimoto, head of the Kumamoto Prefecture Planning Department, and Mr. Shido, head of the prefecture's Pollution Countermeasures Office, when they were here [in Tokyo] was a proposal produced by the company.

AGUNE: In other words, what you handed them was drafted not by the ministry but by the company?

MUTO: That is correct.

The three men named by Muto had petitioned the ministry to establish a mediating body. When he received the document from Muto, Yamada phoned the Minamata city office, dictated the document, and had it presented to the Mutual Aid Association. After the paper was signed, the Committee for Dealing with Minamata Disease Compensation was established. Headed by Tatsuo Chikusa of the Ministry of Labor's Central Labor Relations Commission, the committee also included Shigeo Miyoshi, vice-chairman of the Local Government System Research Council, and Akira Kasamatsu, a professor in Tokyo University's Faculty of Medicine. Every attempt was made to disseminate the view that the committee represented the state and was the appropriate body to entrust with the problem. A public-relations campaign was conducted to persuade people that this prestigious committee would ensure fair compensation.

The seemingly monolithic Mutual Aid Association buckled under the pressure. Some patients were deluded into believing that the Compensation Committee was their best bet, and consequently the association was divided into a faction in favor of fighting Chisso in court and a faction advocating mediation. Members of the latter group, duped into accepting a document based on a draft prepared by Chisso, had once again been maneuvered into a corner, as in 1959 when the "condolence gift" agreement had been forced on patients.

This time, however, circumstances were different in one important respect: a number of patients clearly understood the true nature of the enemy. Resolved to avenge the innocent dead, whatever the cost, they were determined to file suit against Chisso. This group enjoyed the not inconsiderable support of the Association to Indict and the Citizens' Council.

On June 14, 1969, thirteen years after the first patients had been officially identified, twenty-nine families (112 people) filed suit against Chisso with the Kumamoto District Court, demanding a total of ¥640 million in compensation.

Eizo Watanabe, seventy, represented the plaintiffs. His wife had suffered from Minamata disease for twelve years, only to die four months before the suit was filed. The old man felt he had to win the case to enable her spirit to rest in peace. Though winning would not lessen his grief at her loss, he was determined to join battle with a government that consistently protected wrongdoers and in this way expose Chisso's callous attitude toward human life. The battle would be the crowning achievement of his life.

"We are prepared to challenge the authority of the state!" he declared defiantly. "The national government has connived with local authorities to keep us down and to make everyone think Minamata disease is over and done with. But it's not. This year alone, my wife and our friend [Susumu] Sugimoto have died of it. We'll avenge their deaths by winning this case. The company is sure to use its money and authority against us. We must be ready to keep fighting, no matter how long it takes!"

Watanabe was a pillar of strength to the plaintiffs and their supporters, who tended to vacillate. But many Minamata citizens were subservient to Chisso and harshly criticized his efforts. They said he was crazy to take the company to court and condemned the plaintiffs' demand for ¥13 million compensation for each death as exorbitant. In addition, they warned, if the trial brought about Chisso's collapse it would mean the end of Minamata, as well. "Who is more important," they asked, "Minamata's population of fifty thousand or a hundred-odd patients?"

7. THE MAY 25 ACTION

THE MARCH 5, 1970, issue of the newspaper *Mainichi Shimbun* reported that the Compensation Committee had proposed the following payments: ¥2 million for a death and annuities ranging from ¥140,000 to ¥300,000 for living patients. When they heard this, the patients who had put their trust in the committee shook their heads in disbelief. How could the committee suggest such low figures? It must be a rumor spread by Chisso to test the patients' reaction.

Soliciting comment for the journal *Kokuhatsu*, Michiko called on sixty-four-year-old Akino Nagashima, who had lost her husband to the disease. She lived in poverty near Chisso's waste outlet into Hyakken Harbor. Asked for her reaction to the committee's proposal, Akino said, "The committee members think a life can be bought for two million yen. If they really think so, why don't they sell their own lives for that price? They're supposed to be so grand, but look at the way they treat us over compensation. They must think human beings are worth no more than insects."

Akino's husband, Tatsujiro, had been a handsome, husky man. He had been a model worker at the Chisso plant. One day in 1944 nitric acid accidentally gushed out of a pipe, covering him from head to foot and burning his entire body. When Akino rushed to the plant upon being notified, her husband was more dead than alive. His face was so swollen it was impossible to distinguish his features. Nursed assiduously by Akino, he underwent a series of operations to separate his nose from his lips, to open his eyes, and to separate his chin from his chest.

Three years later, still horribly disfigured, he left the hospital. After that he stayed at home, avoiding people as much as possible. His sole pleasure was night fishing. The fish he caught went well with the sakè he loved. Ultimately, however, he fell victim to Minamata disease. Once again life became a round of suffering for Akino. Tatsujiro died on July 9, 1967. For twenty of their forty years together, Akino had been his nurse.

Akino Nagashima's lament that the authorities thought human beings no better than insects reminded Michiko of the famous dictum of Shitagau Noguchi, Chisso's founder. When the firm was about to open a plant in Korea, Noguchi called his employees together and, exhorting them to increase production, said, "Don't think of factory workers as people. Think of them as cattle and treat them like cattle."

This attitude became the norm in Chisso factories. If Chisso regarded its own workers as cattle, it is scarcely surprising that it rated the lowly Minamata-disease patients as mere insects. After all, it was the company's lack of concern for human beings that had led it to pump mercury into the Shiranui Sea at a steadily accelerating rate for the sake of greater productivity. Testimony like the following, delivered during the trial in the Kumamoto District Court by former factory workers, attests to the company's callousness.

Masaharu Eguchi, former labor-union official: Both before and after World War II there was a rigorously implemented system of discrimination between office employees and factory workers. Employees were paid monthly salaries; factory workers were paid by the day. An employee's bonus was the equivalent of three or four months' salary; a factory worker received the equivalent of five days' pay. Factory workers were forbidden to use the employees' cafeteria. Employees wore silver badges, while factory workers wore lead badges three times as heavy as the silver ones. The discrimination prevailing within the company carried over into the community and infected children's attitudes. Factory-worker trainees were called "boy" and were forced to run errands for employees' wives. On one occasion, an employee's wife told a trainee she had something important for him to deliver to the company. The "something important" was a stool specimen she wished to submit for examination.

Shinzo Ogata, former security employee: In 1961 an accidental explosion killed four people. My face was so badly burned that I stayed home swathed in bandages. In fact, I had been told to stay home to avoid the messy situation that would arise if the Labor Standards Bureau noticed occupationally related injuries. We were ordered not to report accidental explosions to the fire department or the police. Explosions make a lot of noise. If neighbors telephoned to inquire about them, we were supposed to say nothing had happened. Fire trucks weren't allowed into the plant grounds; they were turned away at the gate.

Hajime Tanoue, former worker in the acetic acid plant: Ordinarily we used twelve kilograms of mercury in eight hours, but to speed up production sometimes we'd use a kilogram in ten minutes. To make room for new base solution, we'd drain off and dispose of as much as two tons of old base solution in eight hours. Vats containing scrap iron were supposed to extract the mercury from the old base solution, but they were useless because the iron dissolved so fast.

Michiaki Cho, former worker in the acetic acid plant: On the company's entrance examination, we were asked whether we were prepared to die if acetic acid blew up, as it sometimes did. After I was hired, I learned just how dangerous acetic acid is. New clothes were rags the second day they were worn on the job. In the summer we worked in nothing but loincloths. We all had skin problems from the steam and foam of the base solution. There were a lot of explosions during my years there, between 1950 and 1962. The hydrogen chloride gen-

erator blew up the most. There were more than ten such accidents while I was on duty. A big explosion occurred in 1957,
when they were installing a new generator. I got glass and
carbon all over my face. A piece as big as a soybean is still
embedded. The safety valve just didn't work. When I retired,
I considered myself lucky to have survived. The liquid waste
we dumped was never analyzed in the plant.

The May 4, 1970, issue of the *Nishi Nippon Shimbun* published
new information on the Compensation Committee's proposal:
living patients were now to be paid ¥164,000 to ¥320,000 a year,
and a maximum of ¥3 million was to be paid to compensate a
death. If a patient had signed the 1959 "condolence gift" agreement, the sum received at that time would be deducted from
the payment. The committee was to announce its decision to the
patients and Chisso on May 25. The Association to Indict responded with a written protest:

> To all our friends throughout the country who are bound to-
> gether by *Kokuhatsu:* On May 25 the Committee for Dealing
> with Minamata Disease Compensation will notify the patients
> who have agreed to accept its mediation of the compensation
> figures it proposes.
>
> To decide that an organization that has driven people to
> insanity and death out of sheer greed shall pay compensation
> of only ¥3 million for loss of life is beyond belief. But the most
> criminal feature of the committee's proposal is its failure to
> establish Chisso Corporation's responsibility.
>
> The committee's failure in this regard is clearly revealed in
> its mention of the "condolence gift" agreement of 1959. That
> agreement has become the focus of great resentment because
> it was forced on the patients and was based on the desire to
> absolve Chisso of responsibility. The Compensation Com-
> mittee is now attempting to force through its decision, just as
> the "condolence gift" agreement was forced through. The

committee, in collusion with Chisso, is trying to legitimize the attitude underlying that agreement.

Chisso bears criminal responsibility for at least 70 percent of Minamata-disease patients. We have joined forces with the twenty-nine families that have rejected the Compensation Committee's mediation and decided instead to take the matter to court. Accepting the committee's proposal would be tantamount to betraying these people. Nevertheless, there is no real distinction between the patients favoring a trial and those favoring mediation. We cannot allow those who have opted for mediation to be ruined.

Friends throughout Japan, we warn you that the present situation threatens to lead to a repetition of the bitter circumstances of 1959. What would you have done if you had been there at the time? This is the question confronting us.

Friends, the time has come to put our all into the battle to prevent the Compensation Committee from enforcing its proposal. What is needed now is not a mere show of opposition but the resolution and action to bring this course of events to a halt.

The profound resentment and hatred the fishing people of Minamata feel for Chisso must find expression on May 25. We have to make the Chisso management and the Compensation Committee realize that they must repay the blood debt. The Association to Indict [Those Responsible for] Minamata Disease will put its life on the line on May 25.

As the day of the announcement approached, patients, accompanied by friends from the Citizens' Council and the Association to Indict, set out for Tokyo, where they would join other sympathizers determined to help them try to prevent the committee from announcing its proposal. Michiko was among the Minamata contingent. Her son, Michio, then a student at a university in Nagoya, also traveled to Tokyo to be with her.

At 8:00 A.M. on May 25, about 120 people gathered in Tokyo's Hibiya Park, not far from the building housing the Health and Welfare Ministry. Some carried placards bearing enlarged photographs of seriously affected patients. On their chests they bore other placards with such slogans as "Say no to the phony compensation proposal!" and "Forty-five dead Minamata patients are watching today!"

Keikichi Honda addressed the demonstrators: "Today the Compensation Committee is going to try to play out the farce dreamed up by Chisso. After polluting the beautiful sea of Minamata and tormenting the local fishing population, Chisso has consistently deceived us all. We won't stand for it!"

Jun Ui cried out, "We'll fight with all our might! We must put a stop to thirty-four years of collusion between Chisso and the state!"

Michiko bore a placard with a photograph of Tsurumatsu Kama, one of the first Minamata-disease patients she had seen. Watching his mother hold the picture of the wasted old man as if it were a precious relic, Michio was pierced to the heart. His mother had used her pen to describe these stricken people almost as long as he could remember; he had watched as her efforts spread from remote Minamata, ultimately inspiring a united front capable of shaking the nation's capital.

At 9:00 the demonstrators began moving solemnly toward the ministry, where the Compensation Committee was to announce its decision. The ministry had shut the steel gate to the compound. Behind the gate stood grim-faced guards, flanked by men who seemed to be security personnel.

Cries of protest, led by Honda, echoed through the streets: "Open up! Let us see the Compensation Committee! You call yourselves the Ministry of Health and Welfare, but you shut out poor citizens!"

The guards stepped back before the sea of photographs of patients. Shouts of "Who has done this to us? Who are you protecting?" stopped ministry officials in their tracks. Taking advantage of the momentary confusion, sixteen people clambered over the gate, dashed into the building, and headed for the fifth-floor conference room in which the committee was meeting. Thrusting his head out a window, Ui called to the demonstrators below, "We've taken the meeting room!" Noriaki Tsuchimoto, director of numerous documentary films on Minamata disease, added that they would now read a message of protest to the committee. Gazing up at the fifth-floor windows, Michiko and the others waiting outside broke into applause.

Those who had occupied the conference room organized a sit-down blockade of the door, letting in only members of the press. Then they began reading their appeal to the Compensation Committee. Behind a human wall of reporters and photographers, ministry officials ordered the demonstrators blocking access to the room to leave at once, but they only tightened their ranks. A ministry employee who disagreed with the ministry's policies opened a window and warned those waiting outside, "The police are standing by and are ready to use force."

At 9:45 the ministry and the Compensation Committee called in the police to clear the demonstrators from the conference room. The protesters, outnumbered four to one, were pulled and shoved down the stairs. Thirteen people, including Ui and Tsuchimoto, were arrested. Honda, in the forefront of those gathered outside the ministry, called out, "The Ministry of Health and Welfare ought to change its name! You protect Chisso and torment its victims. To stand by now is to collude with Chisso in its criminal enterprise. You'll all be accomplices to murder. Change the ministry's name!"

The demonstrators could hardly believe their ears when they heard that the committee had now announced ¥3.5 million as the maximum compensation for loss of life. They shouted angrily to the windows above, "Is life that cheap in Minamata?" They became more and more enraged as further information filtered out. They learned that the patients' representatives had flatly rejected the committee's proposal; that the mayor of Minamata and the head of the Minamata Fishermen's Cooperative had tried to persuade the representatives to accept the committee's settlement; that ministry officials had done their best to keep the representatives from having any contact with outsiders.

That evening detectives loaded the thirteen arrested demonstrators, still handcuffed, into two patrol wagons in the ministry compound to take them to a nearby police station. Demonstrators formed a human barricade to block egress. The wagons headed for another exit but found it barred by fifty or so students. "Call the riot police!" a hysterical voice cried out. As if awaiting that summons, riot police arrived and swiftly began clearing the area of demonstrators. Some of the students fell back enough to allow the patrol wagons to pass through. Suddenly a young man dashed into the street and, arms outspread, leaped in front of the leading wagon. A detective shouted at the driver to ignore him and keep going. Jumping aside at the last moment, the student narrowly escaped death. The wagons sped off toward the police station. Despite the arrests, the rest of the group continued demonstrating into the night.

The front page of the evening edition of that day's *Asahi Shimbun* newspaper reported that the Compensation Committee had offered ¥3.5 million as compensation for death from Minamata disease and had set annuities for living patients at ¥170,000 to ¥380,000. The paper also gave prominent coverage to another case in which, the same day, maximum compensation of ¥19 million had been agreed on for victims killed in a gas explosion in Osaka. What a difference in the valuation of human life!

In a related story on its human-interest page that evening, the *Asahi Shimbun* quoted Michiko as saying, "I realize that some of the patients who agreed to abide by the Compensation Committee's decision will feel obliged to accept this offer, since the Ministry of Health and Welfare had them sign a statement giving the committee carte blanche. It is painfully clear now that the matter should have been taken to court."

Some people within the ministry were deeply moved by the events of May 25. The next day, a group of staffers sympathetic to the protesters distributed handbills appealing for acknowledgment of the ministry's own responsibility for Minamata disease. This was the first time an internal condemnation of the ministry's policies had ever occurred. The handbill read in part:

> What is the meaning of yesterday's events? The Committee for Dealing with Minamata Disease Compensation announced

its proposal. Ministry personnel were ordered to block all entrances to the building. The ministry, which should be open to all as the guardian of national health and welfare, closed its doors.

Why did we permit the authorities to take this attitude toward the members of the Association to Indict [Those Responsible for] Minamata Disease and their just objections to their lot? In whose behalf are we engaged in social-security work? These questions demand answers.

Although employed by the Ministry of Health and Welfare, we knew far too little about Minamata disease. But yesterday we saw and heard for ourselves how the ministry authorities were conspiring with big business to isolate and conceal the victims.

Fellow ministry employees, Minamata disease has imposed on us a heavy burden that we must carry the rest of our lives. We must not avert our eyes from the pollution within our own ministry.

Let us, having been accused of complicity by the Minamata-disease patients, join forces with our accusers and take a hard look at the irregularities occurring around us. Let us read the account in Michiko Ishimure's *Paradise of the Bitter Sea* of the inhuman conditions caused by pollution and the illness arising from it and thus reinforce our sense of solidarity with the victims so that we can act in their behalf.

The ministry authorities were shocked to learn that some of their own underlings had distributed handbills exposing the seamy side of the government welfare establishment. Michio Hashimoto, director of the ministry's Pollution Division, issued the following statement:

We consider the compensation proposal presented yesterday to be the best possible within the framework of the present system. It is highly regrettable, in view of the regulations governing national civil servants, that members of the ministry staff should have initiated opposition activities.

To this the staff members involved replied:

"The best possible within the framework" is nothing but an evasive figure of speech. The May 25 action was an indictment of thinking in terms of frameworks. Our own actions were entirely in keeping with the spirit of the regulations governing civil servants, who are charged to serve the people. If he considers this regrettable, the director of the Pollution Division should resign and go to work for Chisso. Fellow ministry employees, the Minamata-disease problem will be with us for a long time to come. We urge you not only to make contributions to assist those patients who wish to take the matter to court but also to learn to see their problem as your own by reading their publication *Kokuhatsu.*

Although the authorities had summoned representatives of the patients to travel all the way from Minamata to Tokyo, when the representatives refused to agree to the Compensation Committee's proposal they were shut up in a room in the ministry and forbidden to see any newspapers. After three days of virtual imprisonment, with nothing but box lunches to eat, they were confronted with further cause for grief. The May 27 evening edition of the *Asahi* carried the headline "Agreement Reached on Minamata Compensation: Maximum Raised by ¥500,000." A related story on the human-interest page bore the headline "Conciliatory Patients Crushed; Health and Welfare Ministry, Chisso All Smiles."

The morning edition of the May 28 *Asahi* published a dialogue among Tsutomu Minakami, a writer; Yoshihiro Nomura, professor of law at Tokyo Metropolitan University; and Tatsuo Chikusa, chairman of the Compensation Committee. The headline was "Is This What Minamata Lives Are Worth?" The following excerpt reveals the Compensation Committee's contempt for victims of Minamata disease.

MINAKAMI: Mr. Chikusa, how would you like it if someone decided your life was worth only four million yen?

CHIKUSA: I don't want anyone deciding my life is worth either four million or ten million yen. The point is, I don't think you can ask a person to pay unless that person's responsibility has been clearly established. . . .

NOMURA: No distinction should be made among human lives in either legal or moral settlements. In this case, in which moral considerations should have been paramount, the settlement was too low.

MINAKAMI: I agree entirely.

CHIKUSA: But what would have happened if the company had refused to agree to mediation? On what basis do you claim that the settlement is too low?

NOMURA: Today ten million yen is considered the standard compensation for loss of life.

CHIKUSA: Why should today's standard be applied to something that happened over a decade ago? . . .

MINAKAMI: Was the figure based on the company's suggestion? The committee could have tried to raise the figure, couldn't it?

NOMURA: Couldn't a settlement closer to the norm in terms of both moral and social responsibility have been worked out?

CHIKUSA: The value of money in Minamata is different from what it is in Tokyo. In this case, the minimum annual compensation is one hundred seventy thousand yen. People who aren't seriously incapacitated will receive their wages as well. Actually, the compensation seems too high to me.

The *Asahi* had asked Michiko to take part in the discussion, but she had refused. She despised the committee for pretending to be impartial while offering a pittance for human lives and arresting innocent people for opposing injustice. She had no intention of sitting down with people who could perpetrate such a sham.

Shortly after the stormy events of May 25, a Tokyo chapter of the Association to Indict was formed. Chapters had been springing up around the country among readers of *Paradise of the Bitter Sea*, but the establishment of a foothold in the capital was especially encouraging and represented the fulfillment of one of Michiko's most cherished dreams.

On June 28 the new chapter was formally inaugurated at a gathering of about eight hundred people in a large lecture room in the Department of Urban Engineering at Tokyo University, where Ui taught. Other organizers included Ryutaro Takagi, a producer of films on Minamata disease, and Akira Sunada, a playwright and leader of a theater troupe. Eizo Watanabe, representative of the twenty-nine families that had filed suit against Chisso in June 1969, traveled from Minamata to Tokyo for the occasion. He was accompanied by Michiko and by Fumiko Hiyoshi of the Citizens' Council.

Expecting a modest gathering of forty or fifty people at most, they were moved to see hundreds assembled to greet them. A wave of applause swept through the room as Watanabe stepped to the lectern. Gripping the text of his remarks in trembling hands, he said, "Heaven helps those who help themselves. We victims of Minamata disease are doing our best in the battle against the authorities, but we can't win without your support. Since you might tire if you thought the battle was entirely for the sake of others, make it your own battle, too."

Once again applause thundered through the room. Ui was overcome by emotion as he recalled his own long struggle to force those responsible for Minamata disease to pay for their wickedness, working with Michiko to identify patients and writing about the disease under a pseudonym. His efforts to combat the excesses of modern civilization, which in putting science ahead of all else was driving humanity to the brink of destruction, seemed finally to have struck a chord of sympathy in others. He called out, "We'll follow the patients to the depths of hell! That's the true Minamata struggle!"

8. PILGRIMS AND PILGRIMAGES

MICHIKO'S BOOK changed the lives of many people by drawing them into the world of Minamata-disease patients. One such person was Akira Sunada, head of the theater troupe Chikyuza. He obtained a copy of *Paradise of the Bitter Sea* in 1970 and read it in a single sitting, deeply moved by its vision of hell on the shores of the gleaming Shiranui Sea. Eager to do something to help the patients, he began to think about dramatizing the book. Performing such a play throughout Japan, he thought, might help awaken people to the peril of the scientific civilization that had bewitched so many people. He hoped ultimately to take the play to Minamata itself. But since a project of this kind would take time and entail careful preparation, he decided to put it off for a while in favor of some action that would have a more immediate impact. He finally decided to embark on a fund-raising pilgrimage from Tokyo to Minamata.

Sunada's original plan was to travel alone. But when he discussed the idea with her, Michiko suggested that he organize a group of sympathetic people to walk with him through major cities, soliciting funds to aid the patients. She also suggested that, since Minamata was a sacred place to those involved in the cause, white Buddhist-pilgrim clothing would be the most appropriate attire. Perhaps she was recalling the white robes and plaintively tinkling bells of the pilgrims she had seen walking beside the azure waters of the Shiranui Sea when she was a child.

Realizing that group participation would make his campaign

more effective, Sunada persuaded nine young people to join him. Some were university students; others were members of his troupe. On July 3, 1970, the ten pilgrims, wearing white robes and broad-brimmed straw hats and carrying alms bags, met in front of Chisso's Tokyo headquarters in the midtown Marunouchi business district. Seen off by members of the newly formed Tokyo chapter of the Association to Indict, they set forth.

As they walked along, their shouted demand that Chisso acknowledge its responsibility for Minamata disease echoed from the office buildings. The goodwill with which people placed donations in their alms bags was touching. A day laborer handed over his entire wallet. A child gave pocket money just received from a parent. A housewife donated money with which she had intended to buy food for the evening meal. The pilgrims bowed their heads to each donor and brought their palms together in gratitude, vowing that all the money received would be faithfully transferred to victims of the disease.

On July 9 the pilgrims arrived in Kumamoto City, where they were to attend a meeting of patients and patients' families in support of the trial then underway in the Kumamoto District Court. Members of the Citizens' Council and the Association to Indict, the two major support organizations, as well as representatives of the patients met the pilgrims' train. Three hundred patients and family members awaited the group in the hall of a building in midtown Kumamoto. Thunderous applause greeted the pilgrims when they entered the hall. As part of the opening formalities, sakè was poured, and Fumiko Hiyoshi and Keikichi Honda led the assembly in toasting the cause. Then, asking the patients to accept what they had brought, the pilgrims emptied their alms bags on the speaker's platform. Coins clattered and bills fluttered onto the white cloth spread on the floor. Announcement of a total of ¥653,144 silenced the hall. Rushing to the platform, the patients gazed in awe at the money. Some began sobbing.

The next day, the pilgrims took part in a march in support of those fighting in court. Then they headed for Minamata, their final destination. When they first saw the Shiranui Sea from the train windows, it was wreathed in rain and mist. Everyone in the group recalled passages from *Paradise of the Bitter Sea*. Who would have thought that deadly organic mercury lurked at the bottom of this gentle-looking body of water?

Relieved to have delivered their money safely into the hands of the patients, all were absorbed in their own thoughts. Sunada, who had been sitting with his eyes closed, suddenly opened them. Their pilgrimage must not be allowed to end as a mere sentimental journey, he resolved. Indeed, their pilgrimage had just begun; a long, hard road stretched before them. He recalled Eizo Watanabe's words: "Since you might tire if you thought the battle was entirely for the sake of others, make it your own battle, too." On reaching Minamata, the pilgrims went to Michiko's house, where they removed the soiled white garments they had worn throughout their journey and conducted a ceremony to mark its conclusion.

Sunada completed the script of the play *Paradise of the Bitter Sea* the following year and once again traveled from Tokyo to Minamata, giving performances along the way in what he called his "Bitter Sea pilgrimage." Eventually he moved to the hamlet of Yudo. Living in a small house on a hill overlooking Fukuro Bay and the Amakusa Islands, he and his wife blended into the local population. He became deeply involved in the affairs of the patients through the work of his new troupe, Shiranuiza, and through his quarterly publication, *Shiranui*.

The internationally known American photojournalist W. Eugene Smith learned of Minamata disease through an English translation of the chapter of *Paradise of the Bitter Sea* titled "Yuki's Testimony." Michiko's eloquent evocation of the patients' suffering made such an impression on him that he decided to live in Minamata for a while to compile a photographic record of the disease. Fifty-two years of age at the time, he arrived in Japan in August 1971 with his wife, Aileen. She, of Japanese descent and twenty years his junior, served him as both assistant and interpreter. They rented a farmhouse in the hamlet of Tsukinoura, where there was a high incidence of the disease, and set to work.

In addition to familiarizing himself with the patients and their circumstances by reading Aileen's translations of Michiko's writings, Eugene Smith made a deliberate effort to adapt to the patients' way of life, believing that he could accurately reflect the minds and hearts of his subjects only by living in the same world. Accompanied by Aileen, he would walk along the shore, calling at patients' houses. He was a perfectionist who took picture after picture until he was fully satisfied, but he always held back if he sensed the slightest reluctance on the part of a subject. He never began shooting unless he had the subject's full understanding and consent. Aileen conveyed his feelings to the patients, carefully interpreting everything he said. Understandably, the people he encountered considered him much more thoughtful than most Japanese photojournalists, who were ruthless in their pursuit of the perfect picture.

Eugene found the plight of children congenitally afflicted with the disease particularly distressing. One such child was Tomoko Kamimura, who though well into her teens was totally helpless. Her thin, twisted arms and legs were rigid. She seemed devoid of feeling and perception. A pathetic "Ah!" was the only sound she could make. But her parents had refused to commit her to an institution. She was their special treasure, they said, and they devoted themselves to her care.

Her mother, Yoshiko, was so fond of fish and shellfish that she could happily eat them three times a day. But the organic mercury in the seafood she had eaten while pregnant with Tomoko had passed through her placenta and concentrated in the body of the unborn infant, leaving the mother unharmed. Thereafter Yoshiko bore other, perfectly healthy children. Because Tomoko's parents regarded her as a sacrificial victim who had drawn all the sickness into herself, they felt a special love for her.

Eugene wanted to photograph Yoshiko holding her daughter, but for some time he was too blinded by tears to focus his camera. Eventually, however, he controlled himself sufficiently to take the photograph that became a symbol of Minamata disease. In a dimly lit bathroom, Yoshiko is bathing her daughter. The girl stares with vacant eyes. The mother's face, turned toward her deformed child, glows with love. Eugene's soul went into this photograph, which shocked the world when it appeared in *Life* magazine.

Shinobu Sakamoto was another congenitally afflicted child whom Smith photographed. Shinobu, also in her teens, was more fortunate than Tomoko. She could walk haltingly, and though her speech was slurred, she could make herself understood. Despite her disabilities, every day she had her mother dress her in the uniform of navy blue skirt and sailor blouse worn by Japanese middle school girls and managed to attend special classes for the handicapped.

Eugene made a full photographic record of Shinobu's daily life, while Aileen encouraged her to express her thoughts and feelings. Owing to the girl's speech impediment and to the local dialect she spoke, Aileen often had to ask her the same question over and over. But ultimately she pieced together the following testimony:

> Even when I was little, lots of times I wanted to die because I couldn't run like the others. Because of the way I am I can't ever get married. Mother and father take care of me now, but when they die I'll be all alone. When my brother gets married I'll be a burden. I can't forgive Chisso for doing this to me. Even if we win the trial, I won't get any better, so what difference does it make? What good will the money be? I want them to give me legs and a voice like yours.

In 1973 Eugene's photographs of this girl who strove to live as normally as possible despite her handicaps were published by the Japanese publisher Sojusha in book form, together with a text by Michiko. Their joint effort was titled *Hana-boshi* (Flower Hat), the name Michiko had given to Shinobu's favorite hat.

The Smiths loved Minamata and would have been willing to settle there. But in January 1972, when Eugene was photographing a demonstration at Chisso's plant in Goi, Chiba Prefecture, some Chisso employees assaulted him, inflicting head injuries that threatened his sight. In 1973 he was forced to return to the United States for treatment; and so he and Aileen bade Minamata farewell.

What a strange way to begin an annual shareholders' meeting, thought Michiko as she entered the auditorium of the Kosei Nenkin Building in Osaka on November 28, 1970, in the wake of a group of Minamata-disease patients and patients' families. Wearing white pilgrim garb and carrying memorial tablets of dead family members, they filed past rows of Chisso guards and menacing professional fixers, called *sokaiya*, who intimidated corporate executives into hiring them to keep shareholders under control at shareholders' meetings.

To confront Chisso's president and force the corporation to admit its responsibility, the patients had carried out a campaign to buy single shares and thus obtain the right to attend the shareholders' meeting. Purplish smoke rose from the incense burners some members of the group held in their hands. From the railing of the auditorium's balcony hung banners bearing the Chinese character *on* (rancor) written in white on a black ground. Michiko herself had made the banners to symbolize the bitter memory of the agonizing deaths of Minamata-disease patients.

A voice called for a silent prayer for the dead. A hush fell over the hall and everyone rose. The pilgrims began to chant:

> "Though we think this world
> One long spring,
> It is really only a fleeting dream.
> Before your departed souls we offer
> Sincere and scalding tears and
> Remember you in sorrow."

In the stillness following the chant, a voice rang out: "Hear the rancor the Minamata-disease patients have harbored for the past seventeen years!" Resentment seemed to hang frozen in the air. Thinking back on the long history of oppression she had witnessed, Michiko felt her heart chill.

The curtain concealing the stage now rose to reveal a long table, covered with a white cloth, at which sat a group of Chisso executives with the president, Yutaka Egashira, in the center. He slowly stood.

Suddenly a woman seated directly in front of Michiko rose, clutching memorial tablets of her dead parents in her trembling hands, and cried out, "Murderers! Murderers!" She had lost both parents to the disease, and it had deformed her younger brother. She glared at the stage. Egashira blanched at this unexpected development. The executives glanced at the fixers seated in the first row. One executive said, "In accordance with the corporate regulations, are there no objections?" "No objections! No objections!" called out the fixers. And the curtain began to descend briskly—only four minutes after the meeting had begun.

"Objection! I have an objection!" shouted a lawyer for the patients, leaping onto the stage. As if his shout were a signal, members of the Association to Indict dashed onto the stage, followed by white-clad patients. The company banners at the sides of the stage were torn down, and the white tablecloth was ripped away. Michiko joined the people on the stage, where members of the Association to Indict were surrounding the patients as if to protect them from the Chisso guards. The ringing of pilgrims' hand bells was reinforced by Buddhist chants.

Egashira tried to leave the stage but was stopped by members of the Association to Indict and dragged back to confront the patients. These members, who had gathered for the occasion from all over Japan, formed a living wall around the president and his accusers and, remaining in the background themselves, made sure the patients occupied center stage.

Memorial tablets in hand, the patients turned on the president. Following is an abridged record of the verbal assault on Egashira that ensued.

————I lost both my parents. We expect you to treat us in good faith.

EGASHIRA: I am very sorry.

————Bow to the victims. Kneel down! [Egashira sits.]

————Bow to apologize because the shareholders' meeting didn't go the way it should have.

EGASHIRA: Er . . . I am very sorry.

————You know what we're talking about. You can't fool us.

EGASHIRA: That's what I mean. I apologize from the bottom of my heart.

————You don't really mean that.

EGASHIRA: Yes, I do.

————No, you don't! What right have you to be alive? Die! That's the best way to make amends.

EGASHIRA: I do apologize . . .

————You think life can be bought with money, don't you? We're human beings. I've got two patients in my family. One is seven and can't move.

————Here's Eizo Watanabe. He's going to read the apology President Egashira drew up two years ago. Everybody be quiet and listen. [Applause]

[Watanabe begins to read, but his voice is drowned out.]

————What do you mean, pulling the wool over our eyes? I lost my father. You're a father, aren't you? Still you pour poison into the sea and kill other people. You're the murderer who killed my kids.

————Do you realize what you've done?

————Both my parents. Both dead.

[Egashira shrinks back and smiles to hide his discomfiture.]

————There's nothing to smile about. You don't give a damn about human life.

EGASHIRA: From the bottom of my heart . . .

[A woman drops the memorial tablets she has been carrying, and Egashira reaches out to pick them up.]

EGASHIRA: Be careful . . .

————Care? Do you know what care means?

————It seems Mr. Egashira himself is going to read the apology. [Applause] Everybody stand up.

EGASHIRA [reading]: "The Ministry of Health and Welfare has announced that this company is responsible for the pollution causing Minamata disease. I am filled with remorse when I think of the suffering and sorrow to which this has led . . ."

————Cut out the playacting!

————Cry! If you're human enough to have tears to shed.

————Quiet! Michiko Ishimure has something to say. Be quiet and listen to her. [Applause]

MICHIKO: Representatives of the media here today, please cover the proceedings with care and understanding. Please, everyone, return to your seats and leave judgment to heaven. Let's return to our places now.

————Can you understand my feelings? Can you understand how much I've suffered?

MICHIKO: Please, take the patients back to their seats. We can talk about Chisso and its inhuman crimes later. It's time to go.

————Money can't buy a human life. Both parents gone and a brother deformed! People call him a cripple and laugh at him. How are we supposed to go on living? Can you understand what it means for a woman of forty to have supported them for seventeen years? I'll never know what it's like to be married.

EGASHIRA: I understand completely. I genuinely sympathize.

————What goodwill have you ever showed my family? Answer me!

————Mr. Egashira, answer him. I'm a Chisso employee.

————Show us your goodwill!

EGASHIRA: I *am* showing goodwill.

————I'm ashamed to work for Chisso.

MICHIKO: Come now, let's go home.

In response to Michiko's gentle urging, the patients and their supporters departed, like a slowly retreating tide.

The next day, Michiko herself donned white garments and joined a group of patients in a pilgrimage to nearby Mount Koya, a famous temple complex of the ancient Shingon sect of Buddhism and the center of the Kongo style of hymn chanting.

The patients had first started practicing such hymns, and the accompanying bell ringing, for the shareholders' meeting, though their speech impediments and trembling hands made it extremely difficult. Still, they continued to practice doggedly. Michiko wished there were some way to vindicate their naive belief that chanting Buddhist hymns at Mount Koya would have a salutary effect on their illness—the belief that had given rise to the idea of making a pilgrimage there after the shareholders' meeting.

Riding in the swaying bus as it climbed the winding road to Mount Koya, Michiko thought back on the turbulent day they had just spent. After long years of keeping their thoughts to themselves and enduring oppression, the patients had been given the chance to stand up in front of the president of Chisso and, with the support of sympathizers from all over the country, shout out their true feelings.

The weary but tranquil faces of the sleeping pilgrims, lulled by the rocking of the bus, reminded her of the beatific expression worn by ancient statues of the bodhisattva Maitreya. When they are drained of anger and grief, people truly look like bodhisattvas, she thought. Only a day ago these same people had lamented the loss of their loved ones, cried out against their fate, and railed against the president of Chisso. But they were done weeping and now slept peacefully. The Buddhist teaching that one can attain buddhahood in this life seemed true. Contemplating the bodhisattvas around her, Michiko turned her heart toward Mount Koya.

9. Corporate Responsibility

Minamata was first and foremost a company town, and the patients who sued Chisso in June 1969 were defying the city in taking their case to court. Unfortunately, the patients' initial trust in their lawyers was betrayed. The lawyers were ineffectual at best, and to the end they were unable to comprehend the patients' feelings. Michiko was deeply disappointed by the lawyers' lack of zeal, and her disillusionment deepened the gap between the patients and their lawyers. In the end, friends and supporters of the patients actually directed the case.

The plaintiffs went to trial with a formidable legal team of 347 lawyers, the largest ever to be involved in a pollution case. More than 20 of these lawyers were from Kumamoto Prefecture, and another 125 were from Tokyo. But as it turned out, most only lent their names to the cause; the case was actually handled by about 10 lawyers affiliated with the Japan Communist Party.

After the lawyers filed suit on behalf of the plaintiffs on June 14, they issued a strong statement condemning Chisso. It concluded: "In the name of humanity, we vow to fight to the finish to ensure that this will be a fair and just trial that will help bring an end to pollution caused by lack of respect for human life and to policies that place profit above all else." The patients were greatly moved by these words, but they were to learn very quickly that the lawyers would not fulfill their promise. Communication between the plaintiffs and their lawyers began to break down, and Michiko had trouble getting the lawyers even to meet with their clients to discuss the case. She was dumbfounded by one excuse she was given: "We don't have a special telephone line for this case." When she asked the lawyers to defer payment until the trial was over to lessen the burden on the impoverished patients, they complained that the patients played dirty when it came to money. "We've turned away a lot of other clients to concentrate on the Minamata case. The patients should be grateful." It seemed to Michiko and the patients that the lawyers had lost interest when they saw that fighting for the patients' cause was not going to make them any money.

Every effort was made to collect money to pay the lawyers and cut down on expenses. One million yen was scraped together by readers of *Paradise of the Bitter Sea* and other sympathizers, including schoolchildren who gave money earned through part-time jobs; but the money quickly disappeared in meetings and other expenses. Another ¥3 million was donated by Sohyo, the General Council of Trade Unions of Japan, through its Kumamoto Prefecture branch. Members of the Citizens' Council paid out of their own pockets for a car to use for liaison with the patients and worked without pay collecting data and documents for the lawyers. Michiko, known for her dependence on the telephone, paid for all the long-distance calls she made in the patients' behalf and donated all the royalties from her writings to help pay the legal fees. Keikichi Honda of the Association to Indict even went into debt to add a wing to his house for use as an association office. Those who were making such personal sacrifices could not reconcile themselves to the lawyers' "business first" policy. Neither did the lawyers pay much attention to the documents and other materials that the patients and their supporters had gone to so much trouble to collect.

In August the lawyers filed their first brief with the Kumamoto District Court. The patients groaned in disappointment when they read the document, which charged Chisso with violating the Law for Control of Poisonous and Powerful Agents. Unschooled though she was in matters of law, even Michiko could see that this was not enough to establish the enormity of Chisso's negligence or win the court's sympathy. More important, she knew that charging Chisso only with violating this law would not satisfy the patients' long-held dream of exposing Chisso's criminal responsibility for the tragedy of the mercury-poisoned Shiranui Sea and the havoc that had been wreaked on their lives.

The patients' vague unease over their lawyers' attitude quickly escalated to an acute sense of crisis. They could not possibly win their case with such lukewarm representation. Michiko became convinced of the need to set up a new, more widespread support group that would include university researchers and other specialists who could testify in the patients' behalf. She presented her proposal to the Association to Indict at the end of August. Honda agreed with her, and it was decided to create an independent support group to provide legal and medical expertise.

Once the decision had been made, the association moved quickly. Two members in Kumamoto, Nobuo Miyazawa of the Kumamoto bureau of the public radio and television network, NHK, and Kyoji Watanabe, prevailed upon Sadao Togashi, an associate professor in Kumamoto University's Faculty of Law, and Masazumi Harada, an associate professor in the same university's School of Medicine, to come to their aid. Though exhausted by the recent student demonstrations that had disrupted the university, the two agreed to do whatever they could. No one had been sure of their cooperation, and it was with considerable relief that the association welcomed two such powerful allies to the patients' cause.

The two scholars felt a heavy sense of responsibility for the task they had agreed to undertake. They were well acquainted with *Paradise of the Bitter Sea,* and they felt bound to bring Chisso to book for the irreparable harm it had caused. Togashi was critical of the lawyers' brief: "Judging from precedents in negligence cases, it's unlikely that you'd win with this. No attempt has been made to present a solid legal argument against Chisso." Michiko's fears had been confirmed.

An inaugural ceremony to launch the independent support group, named the Minamata Disease Study Group, was held in

Kumamoto City. Those present included Michiko, Togashi, and Harada; Honda, Watanabe, and Miyazawa of the Association to Indict; and Fumiko Hiyoshi of the Citizens' Council.

The Study Group also included four members of the No. 1 Labor Union of Chisso's Minamata plant. This was one of the most remarkable developments in the entire saga of Minamata disease. The union members supplied valuable corporate data that would normally have remained secret, and thus played an important role in turning the case in the patients' favor.

Back in 1959, at the time of the "condolence gift" agreement, the Chisso labor union had sided with management, dismantling the tent the patients had set up at the main entrance to the plant. But in 1962 Chisso had attempted to get the union to agree to a temporary wage freeze, and the ensuing controversy had split the union. Since then the No. 1 Labor Union, which had opposed management, had been discriminated against by the company. For the first time, union members had gained an inkling of the kind of discrimination and prejudice the Minamata-disease patients were subject to. It was this rebel union that supplied the patients with daily manufacturing records and other documents originally destined for the incinerator.

On December 14 Jun Ui, one of the original advocates of taking Chisso to court, addressed the Study Group. After his talk, members of the group and some of the lawyers representing the patients debated the strategy to adopt in the trial. The two groups were at loggerheads from the start, and the atmosphere turned ugly. Togashi asked the lawyers their opinion of the idea that a corporation has a responsibility to ensure safety but received no satisfactory answer. Michiko made no attempt to conceal her disgust with the weak brief prepared by the lawyers even though they had received ¥3 million from Sohyo and documents providing important data painstakingly collected by the patients and their supporters.

The lawyers' inability to reply satisfactorily to the questions of Togashi and Michiko revealed that they had not yet prepared their case. The Association to Indict and the Citizens' Council felt compelled to break off relations with the very lawyers who should have been their allies in the cause. Their incompetence exposed, the lawyers could only sputter, "The Study Group is nothing but a bunch of Trotskyites," as they stomped out of the room. The breach was to remain unhealed up to the day the court handed down its verdict.

The Study Group decided to prepare a research report that would provide a better foundation for the case than the lawyers' first brief. Divided into task groups, the members set about collecting the data they would need, then gathered in a series of overnight sessions led by Harada and Togashi to compare notes and discuss the actual writing of the report. Michiko attended all these meetings, constantly reminding the participants of the immorality of Chisso's disregard of the patients' suffering and of the way in which the company was driving them relentlessly to painful death.

Togashi believed that the report's main objective should be to set forth clearly the patients' complaints and demands. He also felt that it should incorporate Michiko's eloquent testimony and convey her passionate commitment to the patients' cause. Chisso had to be made legally accountable for consigning innocent people to hell. Everyone in the Study Group had first been made aware of the world of the Minamata patients through Michiko's book; it was only fitting, thought Togashi, that the report reflect her perspective.

The completed report, titled "Corporate Responsibility for Minamata Disease: Chisso's Malfeasance," totaled 385 pages. It began with a medical history, in which Harada explained the horrifying effects of Minamata disease on the human body and mind and Michiko painted a compelling portrait of the wretched lives of the patients and their families. The second part of the report was devoted to a review of the cause of Minamata disease and recounted the long-drawn-out process by which the Kumamoto University School of Medicine had traced the cause to organic mercury.

In the third part, Togashi presented his argument of gross corporate negligence. Chisso, he argued, was a typical example of a corporate structure with no regard for safety. Substantiating his argument with facts, Togashi showed that Minamata disease was an inevitable result of corporate irresponsibility. He went on to document the way in which, disregarding safety standards, Chisso had poured untreated poisonous effluent into the Shiranui Sea, then had chosen to ignore the obviously dangerous effects of its action. This argument of corporate negligence was the crux of the patients' case.

The report concluded with a fourth part in which Chisso was charged with willfully neglecting to seek out the cause of Minamata disease after its existence had been officially recognized and with attempting to obstruct Kumamoto University's efforts to pinpoint the cause.

Twenty copies of "Corporate Responsibility" were circulated to various people, including the lawyers on the patients' legal team. Arguing that the report would expose their hand to Chisso, the lawyers asked that the Study Group relinquish its plan to publish the document. The Study Group, however, felt that the legal argument set forth in the report was the only effective weapon against Chisso, and in August 1970 the Association to Indict published five thousand copies.

Another trial involving mercury poisoning was underway in Niigata Prefecture, and copies of the report were sent to the plaintiffs there, as well. On September 29, 1971, the Niigata District Court handed down a ruling against Showa Denko that set a precedent for accepting Togashi's argument of corporate negligence. He was delighted, for now he was confident that the Minamata patients could win their case, as well.

A copy of "Corporate Responsibility" had, of course, been sent to the Kumamoto District Court judge, and as it happened, this was to expose the degree to which the lawyers for the plaintiffs were unwilling to do their own groundwork. The lawyers had branded the Study Group "a bunch of Trotskyites" and had opposed the publication of "Corporate Responsibility." Yet these same lawyers, it was later discovered, plagiarized the research report, misprints and all, in their fourth brief. Not all the lawyers supported this blatant move, and the brief was withdrawn almost as quickly as it had been drawn up. The story of "the brief that never was" soon became a favorite joke among the Study Group members. Despite the lawyers' blundering, the plaintiffs' case in the Kumamoto District Court revolved around "Corporate Responsibility," and Togashi's argument that corporations should be held responsible for gross negligence of public safety was upheld by the court.

Michiko's contribution to this carefully documented report at first seemed strangely out of place. Togashi had asked her to supply an objective, documented, academically precise account of the disease's debilitating effects upon the patients and their families, but what he got was a literary description of the patients' wails of anguish against the cruel assault upon their human dignity. Her writing did not match the rest of the report's carefully objective tone, yet Togashi acknowledged that there was perhaps no other way to convey the patients' suffering. He was well aware of the importance to the plaintiffs' case of Michiko's vision and passionate dedication. He himself had visited the fishing hamlets of Minamata and had met a number of Minamata-disease patients, but they had remained people from another world until Michiko had drawn him into the very depths of the patients' souls. All the members of the Study Group had devoted themselves to the task of compiling the report, but only Michiko's conviction, thought Togashi, could have motivated them so powerfully.

Michiko's writings had a strong impact on the world of medicine, as well. Masazumi Harada had been a member of the Kumamoto University School of Medicine's research team on unusual diseases since 1962. He had seen many cases of congenital Minamata disease. Whenever he examined patients in Minamata, he noticed a woman with bobbed hair sitting in a far corner and intently watching everything he did. At first he assumed she was a district nurse. When their eyes met she would smile faintly, but she never attempted to speak to him. Yet always she was there, watching.

In the mid-1960s, Harada was captivated by a series of essays in the *Kumamoto Fudoki* titled "Between Sea and Sky." This series, a vivid portrayal of the very patients he had been seeing, described their distress in a way that he as a doctor could never have done. Every word reverberated with the patients' soul-deep cries of anguish. No doctor of conscience could ignore their pleas. It was with amazement that Harada learned that the author was the quietly intent woman he had seen when examining patients in Minamata.

Michiko's description of the patients' symptoms was both levelheaded and sympathetic. Harada wondered if he or any other doctor had ever perceived more than the most superficial aspects of patients' condition in making their diagnoses. It is taught in diagnostics that one must listen carefully to what a patient says and must also know quite a bit about the patient's past history and lifestyle. Yet this basic principle was being ignored in the case of Minamata-disease patients. Why did Kumamoto Prefecture's Minamata Disease Patients Screening Board assume that the patients were lying about their condition? Why was Chisso's assertion that their illness was feigned being taken more seriously than the obvious evidence to the contrary? Was it not because, as indicated by patients' frequent outbursts of frustration, doctors paid no attention to their complaints, relying on textbook diagnoses and making no attempt to understand the patients' feelings? Where, in doctors' notes on patients' condition, were the human beings who were suffering? Michiko's essays plagued Harada with such questions.

Harada found the accounts of Minamata-disease patients in "Between Sea and Sky" and, later, *Paradise of the Bitter Sea* far more compelling than any medical records. He began to feel strongly that his own diagnostic records should reflect the same concern and sensitivity, and he bore this in mind when writing the medical histories that would be presented in court. After explaining the complex symptoms of mercury poisoning, he described the details of each patient's life, including such aspects as the patient's physical and emotional responses to societal pressure. He did his best to portray the entire human being.

When those allied with Chisso saw Harada's medical analyses, they complained that they were depositions rather than diagnoses—a reaction that indicated the extent to which specialists, including physicians, had lost touch with the humanity of their subjects. How else could modern medicine have ignored Minamata disease for more than a decade? Fortunately, there were a few doctors who sought to correct this error. Almost all the doctors at the Kumamoto University School of Medicine, which had come to be regarded as the leading authority on Minamata disease, had read Michiko's accounts of the disease. Some believed that only they had the specialized knowledge to understand the disease and disdained her writing as the work of an amateur. Yet others, like Harada, sought to learn from her how to see their patients as human beings with emotions as well as symptoms of disease and worked hard to win their patients' trust.

In "Corporate Responsibility," Harada and Michiko shared equal responsibility for writing about the effects of the disease. It was highly unusual for a lay writer and a physician to collaborate in writing a medical report, but Harada, who had learned from Michiko how to see into the depths of his patients' souls, considered it both natural and right.

In March 1970, when Michiko was busy working on "Corporate Responsibility," she learned that *Paradise of the Bitter Sea* had been selected to receive the first Oya Prize for Nonfiction. Soichi Oya (1900–1970), a sharp-tongued social commentator who had dominated the Japanese media for many years, had established the prize to reward outstanding works of nonfiction. Oya and the jurors had been greatly moved by *Paradise of the Bitter Sea* and were stunned when Michiko refused the prize.

Oya himself had long been suspicious of any claims to social superiority or authority and could not in clear conscience deny that if he had been offered the award, he might well have turned it down, too. He commented wryly, "The famous feminist Itsue Takamure was also from Kumamoto Prefecture. Wouldn't you know there'd be another stubborn woman from that place who'd refuse even my prize." The jurors were not prepared to give up so easily, however. This was, after all, the first Oya Prize. It would not do to have it turned down so summarily. "Please," one of the jurors pleaded to a mutual acquaintance, "tell her even a hard-boiled person like me wept when I read her book. Please persuade her to accept the prize." Representatives of Kodansha, publisher of *Paradise of the Bitter Sea*, also implored Michiko to accept.

No sooner had the news gone out that Michiko's book had been selected for the first Oya Prize than she was inundated by congratulatory messages from supporters all over Japan. She herself, however, was too preoccupied with the trial to pay any attention. Her mother, Haruno, at a loss to respond to all the messages, turned for advice to Kenzo Hashimoto, Itsue Takamure's widower.

"Of course Michiko won't accept any prizes," he said flatly. Haruno agreed. Michiko had been an excellent student as a child, and she had had a fine hand. Haruno remembered how painfully embarrassed Michiko had been when her essays and calligraphy had appeared in the local newspaper. At school, the best examples of calligraphy were displayed where everyone could see them, but Michiko often removed hers. Eventually her father would find her hidden works and proudly display them on a wall at home. Michiko always tore them down, though, muttering angrily, "Why do you put up such calligraphy?" She hated being commended in front of others. She also had a slight stutter and found it painful to speak to groups.

When the Oya Prize selection was announced, Michiko hid for several days. For a while she sought refuge in Chikuho at the home of the writer Hidenobu Ueno, who had proofread *Paradise of the Bitter Sea*. The public clamor would not subside, however, and finally Kyoji Watanabe persuaded Michiko to meet the press.

The reasons Michiko gave for refusing the prize had a certain logic. She did not have the leisure or inclination, she said, to break away from the intense activity surrounding the compilation of "Corporate Responsibility" just to accept recognition for her earlier work. All her energy was concentrated on the trial.

The Oya Prize jury had asked her to write a curriculum vitae, including her literary background, but she had been so busy she had forgotten to do it.

She also felt qualms about being praised for her portrayal of the suffering of Minamata-disease patients. Only because she had thrown in her lot with that of the patients had they come to trust her and open their hearts to her. She could not neglect them now just to receive a prize. Another concern was the effect her acceptance of the prize would have on public opinion in Minamata. Critics were certain to charge that she had used the Minamata patients to serve her own ends. It would be harder than ever for her family to continue living in Minamata.

In 1969, when *Paradise of the Bitter Sea* was published, a group of friends led by Ueno had gone to Michiko's house to offer their congratulations. Her father had asked worriedly, "How is the book being received outside Minamata?" He knew how the people of Minamata resented his daughter for her involvement with the patients and how they harassed her for her dedication. Aware of how risky it was to defy Chisso in this provincial city, he was concerned about the way her book was being received elsewhere. Ueno reassured him: "Michiko has done something not even a man could have done. Not only did she write a book, but she did it while fighting the patients' battle. Her book has aroused sympathy all over the country." Only when he heard these words was her father able to smile.

The news that *Paradise of the Bitter Sea* had been chosen to receive the first Oya Prize swept through Minamata like wildfire. Especially chagrined by the news were those at Chisso's Minamata plant and the city officials. All their efforts to manipulate public opinion and thus hide the truth about Minamata disease had been in vain. Once again the problem was in the public eye. Uncertain what to do, the city officials continued to obey Chisso directives and studiously ignore the book and its repercussions.

The smallest neighborhood event, the least recognition accorded a Minamata citizen, was described in minute detail in the municipal government's bulletin, but not a line was given to the news of Michiko's book and the Oya Prize. A provincial city like Minamata could not afford to acknowledge the public recognition of one of its own if that meant defying Chisso, on which its very survival depended. But the repudiation of her achievement by the local establishment meant more to Michiko than any literary prize. She had seen the depths of the abyss into which the Minamata-disease patients had been plunged, and worldly honor and fame meant nothing to her.

Oya died unexpectedly the same year. Michiko was shaken by the news, knowing how happy he would have been if she could have brought herself to accept his prize. He had, after all, praised her work highly. The following year the pomelo tree in Michiko's front yard bore fruit for the first time, and she immediately sent one to Oya's widow. Though she enclosed no note, the gift was her way of apologizing for having upset Oya.

10. An Abortive Encounter

THE FISHERS of Minamata have a finely honed sense of justice. Should their child hurt a neighbor's child, they rush over to apologize. If their child accidentally breaks someone's window, it is assumed by one and all that the parents will pay for the damage. Apology and restitution, they firmly believe, are fundamental to justice. In their minds, it was only just that Chisso be held accountable for polluting the Shiranui Sea with mercury and robbing people of their health; no amount of apologizing or financial compensation could be too much.

As Michiko saw it, the least the president of Chisso could do in the name of basic human decency was to visit each of the patients and apologize sincerely for what his company had perpetrated. Yet when the first cases of Minamata disease were identified, the Chisso president studiously avoided meeting the patients. It was not until September 1968, when the central government formally acknowledged that Minamata disease was caused by effluent from Chisso's Minamata plant, that he finally went to patients' homes to apologize. But even this he did only once, and with the greatest reluctance, merely to appease public opinion. There was no sign of sincere remorse. Never did he visit any of the patients later certified.

The gate of the Chisso plant remained tightly closed to newly certified Minamata patients, the Chisso executives rebuffing the patients' demands for a meeting. Michiko was determined to pry the executives out of hiding and force them to meet and talk with the patients. In the spring of 1971, Michiko and Teruo Kawamoto supported the Araki, Isayama, and Chikuchibara families, which included the most recently certified Minamata patients, in their persistent petitions to Chisso for direct negotiations with the president. Chisso finally relented, but insisted that the negotiations be carried out at the Mikasaya inn in Yunoko, a hot-spring resort north of Minamata. The inn was well known as a Chisso haunt. Important company guests were always taken there, and Chisso executives used it as if it were their own villa. The other inns in the area also enjoyed Chisso's patronage. Ironically, the waves washing the beautiful Yunoko coastline were polluted with Chisso's mercury, and some local people had contracted Minamata disease. They were kept hidden away, however, lest visitors be scared away from the resort.

Many years earlier, Michiko's grandfather Matsutaro had directed a project to shore up the Yunoko coastline with stones shipped in from the Amakusa Islands. The Yunoko inns had been built along this waterfront. Some had even purchased the boat Matsutaro had used to haul the stones and converted it into a bath. In a sense, Matsutaro had laid the foundations of a resort that flourished under Chisso patronage and that was now to become Michiko's battleground with the company.

When the patients' family members and representatives, including Michiko, arrived at the Mikasaya on July 3, 1971, they were greeted at the entrance by a contingent of police officers. The inn employees were also on guard, even the proprietor showing up as if to protect the Chisso executives. Since the inn and the hot-spring resort of which it was a part owed their prosperity in large measure to Chisso, it was not surprising that the people of the Mikasaya looked askance at those who dared to challenge Chisso's benevolence.

Chisso's president did not appear, however. On learning of his absence, the pent-up anger and frustration of the patients' families exploded into rage. Exasperated by this turn of events, Michiko, who till then had remained in the background, took the Chisso executives to task: "How can you expect the patients' families to calm down when the president continues to refuse to apologize in person?"

Outside, twilight settled on the Shiranui Sea. The Amakusa Islands were lost in a purple mist. The rippling sea sparkled in the last rays of the setting sun. There was no one to witness this farce of a negotiation, for Chisso had demanded that the local press be kept away.

Representing Chisso were Shoichi Kuga, director of general affairs at the company's Tokyo headquarters; Eiichi Tsuchiya, assistant director of general affairs; Saburo Sasaki, president of the Minamata subsidiary; Isamu Yamane, manager of the Minamata plant; Keiji Higashidaira, director of general affairs at the Minamata plant; and the corporate lawyers Shozo Kusumoto and Yasuhei Tsukamoto. The patients' group comprised family members Ikumatsu and Rui Araki, Shigeru and Reiko Isayama, and Shie Chikuchibara, along with representatives Michiko, Kawamoto, Nobuo Miyazawa, Kimiyo Ito, and the lawyers Akio Manaki, Tetsuya Araki, Sachio Aoki, and Masao Fukuda.

This was the first time since the outbreak of the disease that patients had confronted Chisso with their own representatives. But as Michiko had feared, this first formal meeting only served to expose Chisso's inhuman attitude. The ensuing dialogue indicates the intransigence the patients and their supporters faced.

MANAKI: We ask again: May we meet with the president?

KUGA: We're here to discuss compensation. There's no reason that can't be done by proxy.

RUI ARAKI: An adult doesn't hurt a child and then send a proxy to apologize. You've killed people. Think about that. This isn't something that can be settled by proxy.

KUGA: A company is an organization, and we all have our jobs to do. The president certainly isn't trying to evade the issue by sending us. He feels very keenly for you people.

MANAKI: In that case he should have made every effort to be here today. Has he indicated any intention of seeing us?

KUGA: The next time he comes here [to Minamata].

RUI ARAKI: Is the president sick or something? We're sick, can't even do our work, but we've come. It doesn't matter how many lawyers come. We want to see the boss.

MANAKI: When can the president meet with us? Tell us exactly when he will be available.

HIGASHIDAIRA: I really don't understand what you're driving at. You want both sides to designate representatives to negotiate, but at the same time you say you can't negotiate unless the president is present.

MICHIKO: Isn't it accepted policy in any company for the top person to take responsibility when the company has caused problems? It doesn't make sense to say the president is too busy because he heads a large and complex corporation. These people have left sick family members at home to come here.

CHIKUCHIBARA: You don't even think of us as human beings, do you? We're just animals to you, aren't we?

MANAKI: Back in 1968, when the government officially recognized the disease, your president went around to patients and apologized. Was that an exception? Why isn't he apologizing to the most recently certified patients?

KUSUMOTO: Now, there's no reason to bring up past issues. If you're just out to abuse us, we're going to leave.

MICHIKO: It's not a past issue. The problem is still with us.

MIYAZAWA: These people were just certified.

KUSUMOTO: Let's leave. This is no place for a kangaroo court. [He gathers together the papers on the table and starts to rise.]

KAWAMOTO: We're not trying to abuse anyone. We've just come to make a request.

MANAKI: We're asking if the president has any intention of participating in these negotiations.

HIGASHIDAIRA: Accept us as his representatives. Then we can proceed without him.

MICHIKO: We're not going to make any headway with an attitude like that. The negotiations haven't even started. How can we help doubting your sincerity? That's why we're insisting we want to see the president.

KUSUMOTO: As long as the negotiations can be carried out without the president, there's no need for him to be here.

RUI ARAKI: Look, I'm ready to forget everything else. Just give me back my child well and sound. If she were well, she'd be married and I'd have grandchildren.

IKUMATSU ARAKI: First you strike down innocent people with disease, and now you ask us to agree to some kind of proposal for wrapping up the whole affair. It's not that simple. Like my wife says, the best thing you could do is restore our child to health. More than a hundred people have been certified as Minamata-disease patients so far. Is there even one who has been pronounced fully recovered? As it is, we're raising our daughter only to die. She may live till sixty or die at fifty, who knows? We'll need money, that's for sure.

TSUKAMOTO: The company can't make exceptions.

MICHIKO: What a terrible company Chisso is.

HIGASHIDAIRA: If we don't pay out the amount of money you demand, you say we're terrible. I realize that as patients you can't censure us enough. But condemning us and negotiating compensation are two different things. They don't mix well.

IKUMATSU ARAKI: I bet you haven't been sick since the day you were born. You joined Chisso and you've watched out for the company's interests ever since. I bet you don't know a thing about the suffering of a sick person. You look like a human being, but underneath, you're vermin.

TSUCHIYA: The fact of the matter is, we didn't draw up that compensation proposal on our own. It's the product of careful deliberation by the Compensation Committee.

MANAKI: But you're insisting that the patients accept its terms. You must have your reasons.

KUSUMOTO: We feel that it's generally fair. But we haven't said anything about whether applying its terms to you people is legally valid or not.

MANAKI: It's obviously unfair. The question is, how fair is the amount of money stipulated in your proposal?

TSUKAMOTO: In any case, we haven't considered what is and isn't fair for these people.

MANAKI: Then please consider it.

TSUKAMOTO: We don't see any need to do so. We can't make exceptions. We're asking you to accept the same conditions as everyone else.

MANAKI: Whatever have we come here to talk about, then? There's nothing to negotiate, is there?

KAWAMOTO: You're just forcing your terms on us.

TSUKAMOTO: We're asking you to accept our proposal. If you don't, we have no choice but to break off these talks.

MANAKI: We're here to reach an agreement, aren't we? Agreement means we each have to give up something. But you're insisting right from the start that you can't give up anything. *We* have no choice but to break off the talks.

TSUKAMOTO: Negotiation and agreement are two different things, surely.

MANAKI: Well then, Mr. Kuga. Do you think Chisso is responsible for this disease?

KUGA: That very point is being argued in court right now.

RUI ARAKI: You're saying all kinds of things. Why don't you take our daughter Yasuko. Take her and care for her. I don't ask for anything else. Please, just take her. But then, if you did, you probably wouldn't feed her properly. You'd probably just let her die. As her parents we can't allow that. That's why we're here to talk to you.

CHIKUCHIBARA: Please, I haven't come here to fight. We're fisherfolk, and we're simply trying to pull the net in. That's hard work, and our voices tend to get loud and rough. Please understand.

RUI ARAKI: Why don't we send our sick people to your boss for a month? It's not only the sick who have it hard. It's hard on those taking care of them, too.

KUGA: We do sympathize with you. I know it must be hard for you to accept, but everyone's case is different. We can't treat you all differently.

CHIKUCHIBARA: Different? Everyone's different? That's what you say!

IKUMATSU ARAKI: Why don't you explain the Compensation Committee's position so we can understand?

KUGA: It's all there in the papers we gave you.

MICHIKO: These people aren't used to reading legal documents. We're asking that you explain the situation in language they can understand.

TSUCHIYA: All right. I'll explain it. [He talks for about twenty minutes, explaining the genesis of the Compensation Committee, which was created at the behest of the Ministry of Health and Welfare, and the committee's compensation proposal.]

MIYAZAWA: Chikuchibara was struck down at the peak of his fishing career. He's getting an annuity of a hundred thousand yen. How did you arrive at that figure?

TSUCHIYA: Regarding that point, right now we can't treat him differently from everyone else.

KUSUMOTO: A hundred thousand yen was considered a legally valid amount to cover lost income. The four people certified as Minamata-disease patients last year were treated the same way. The people who have been certified most recently must also expect the same treatment. It's not a question of what's fair or just or acceptable. Those who agreed to rely on mediation were treated that way, so we have to treat you the same way, as I keep saying.

MANAKI: Was a hundred thousand yen ever really enough to live on? Is it because you think it's enough to live on that you're insisting that Araki, Isayama, and Chikuchibara accept that amount?

KUSUMOTO: There's no need to answer that.

CHIKUCHIBARA: You mean a hundred thousand yen a year?

MIYAZAWA: Yes, a year.

CHIKUCHIBARA: Even ten years ago two of us couldn't have lived on a hundred thousand yen a year, even if we ate nothing but pig feed!

FUKUDA: That's less than the government's basic relief allowance was back in 1964, an allowance that was said to be unconstitutional because it didn't permit the "minimum standards of wholesome and cultured living" guaranteed by the Constitution.

CHIKUCHIBARA: You don't see us as human beings, do you? You think of us as animals. Even a pig costs at least a hundred thousand yen a year to feed.

TSUKAMOTO: It doesn't matter how much we discuss it; that's the standard we have to adhere to right now.

CHIKUCHIBARA: You must be made of stone.

KUGA: That's the amount we've offered everyone for years. There's no point debating here whether it's enough to live on or not.

CHIKUCHIBARA: You must think we're fools.

MIYAZAWA: If we accept your annual compensation, we become ineligible for government relief. Did you know that, Mr. Kuga? The patients in Minamata who agreed to mediation have had their relief allowances cut off.

KUGA: That's an administrative problem. There's no point discussing it here.

MANAKI: How do you expect these people to live?

KUGA: We won't get anywhere debating that.

CHIKUCHIBARA: But we have to. That's why we're here.

TSUKAMOTO: I realize you may not be happy with the present arrangements. . . .

MIYAZAWA: It's not a matter of being happy. It's a question of life or death.

KUSUMOTO: Whether you can live on the money is a different issue.

HIGASHIDAIRA: We've accepted a mediation proposal worked out by a third party that's listened to both sides' arguments. It's useless to ask whether it's enough to live on.

CHIKUCHIBARA: I don't know when my sick husband is going to die. And as long as he lives I can't work. Up to now I've felt some obligation to the company. But not anymore.

SHIGERU ISAYAMA: I hear you deducted the amount paid out earlier as "condolence gifts" from the lump-sum payments you made to the people before us.

KUGA: Both sides agreed to that arrangement. The details weren't explained to us, so we can't tell you anything about it.

MIYAZAWA: Even if nothing was explained to you in May 1970, you certainly have an obligation to explain things now to these three families.

HIGASHIDAIRA: If the Compensation Committee had made it clear how it arrived at its proposal, we certainly wouldn't try to hide it. But we didn't draw up the proposal; we left it to the committee.

KAWAMOTO: Are you saying you don't have to explain how you settled on the amount of compensation? That you don't have to give any reasons?

TSUKAMOTO: There's a lot in the compensation proposal that we don't understand.

KAWAMOTO: It's really your own proposal, not the Compensation Committee's, isn't it? So you should be able to explain it. You said yourself the committee's proposal stipulated that it couldn't be applied to patients certified in the future.

HIGASHIDAIRA: I believe such wording appears in any kind of settlement.

MANAKI: You won't explain your reasoning, and you refuse to concede any point. I don't think this can be called negotiating.

HIGASHIDAIRA: If one side says one million yen and the other side says three million yen and then a mediator says one million five hundred thousand yen and we all agree to the final figure, what could be more clear cut than that? After all, the final figure was set by the mediating party.

The Amakusa Islands had faded to a dim silhouette, and the Shiranui Sea was cloaked in dusk. Within the inn, the patients' families and representatives continued to demand to see the Chisso president, while the Chisso representatives continued to refuse. One of the patients' party, an old woman, clung in desperation to a Chisso man as he rose from his seat. He shook her off, and the Chisso representatives stalked out of the room.

Thwarted, the families and friends of the patients resolved, like those before them, to battle Chisso in court.

✧

Shortly after the Mikasaya meeting, the July 12, 1971, issue of the popular weekly magazine *Shukan Bunshun* published excerpts of an interview with a Chisso executive who had ridiculed Minamata-disease patients. He had asserted that Chisso was blameless, that the patients had fallen ill because they had eaten rotten fish and should be grateful they had received any compensation at all. The speaker was Keiji Higashidaira, whose job entailed dealing with the patients and their supporters. *Shukan Bunshun* had quoted Higashidaira's words from the Japanese translation of *Japans harakiri*, by the Swedish reporter Bo Gunnarsson, who had interviewed Higashidaira.

Higashidaira had unwittingly articulated Chisso's true feelings toward the patients, and Chisso officials, worried about the adverse effect his statements might have on their position in the Kumamoto trial, secretly bought up all copies of the magazine distributed in the Minamata area, even subscription copies.

The Kumamoto branch of the Association to Indict had notified the Citizens' Council in advance that Higashidaira's indiscreet remarks were supposed to appear in *Shukan Bunshun*. Eager to get a copy, Satoru Akazaki rose early the day the magazine went on sale and made his way through the morning mist to the newsstand at Minamata Station. But he was already too late. Chisso had got there first, and not a copy was to be found. He rushed to a nearby bookstore, but here too there was no *Shukan Bunshun*. A member of the Citizens' Council had to go all the way to the neighboring prefecture of Kagoshima to obtain a copy. Michiko recalled an acquaintance working for the magazine and with that person's help arranged to have 150 more copies sent immediately.

The Citizens' Council printed leaflets bearing Higashidaira's remarks and had them distributed throughout Minamata as a newspaper insert. The leaflet invited anyone who wanted a copy of the magazine to contact the Citizens' Council. By the end of the day the leaflet appeared, the 150 copies Michiko had obtained were gone. Chisso's attempt to suppress the article had backfired.

Following is an abridged version of Gunnarsson's interview with Higashidaira as published later in *Kokuhatsu* (translated from *Japans harakiri*).

Q: Didn't you think at all of the danger of using mercury?

HIGASHIDAIRA: No, we never tested the mercury to find out if it was poisonous. We knew that the twenty-four other manufacturers of vinyl chlorides had been discharging untreated wastes for a long time with no obvious ill effects. Who would have thought Minamata would be the first case of pollution? We had done everything we thought necessary. It never occurred to us that our effluent was dangerous to humans.

Q: Yet you continued pouring effluent into Minamata Bay even after 1957, when you had some idea that mercury was the cause.

HIGASHIDAIRA: There was no solid proof. Consider: no one got sick after the autumn of 1959, but we installed a special filter anyway. It cost us four hundred million yen. We did everything we could to protect the people of Minamata.

Q: But you acknowledge now that the mercury in Chisso's effluent is the cause of Minamata disease.

HIGASHIDAIRA: There may be a connection. But there are other factors to be considered. For all we know, part of the cause may be some other poisonous substance. There may be something emanating from some other place.

Q: Is there another plant nearby?

HIGASHIDAIRA: No. But since we plan to go into this issue in detail in the trial now underway, I can't comment further.

Q: Didn't Chisso obstruct the efforts of a Kumamoto University team to get samples of effluent from the plant?

HIGASHIDAIRA: That's not true. We just wanted them to give us about a week's notice.

Q: Do you have proof that Chisso is innocent?

HIGASHIDAIRA: Of course. It will be presented at the trial. The truth will come out, and we will be proved innocent. I can't, of course, give you any details right now.

Q: Are the Minamata fishers still eating fish from Minamata Bay?

HIGASHIDAIRA: Yes, and that's an important point. To put it bluntly, they've been eating rotten fish that were floating in the bay. But it's difficult to make this point in court, since it would look as if we were trying to create a bad impression of our opponents. As if they were animals, you know. Those who became sick after 1958, at any rate, should be grateful that they're receiving compensation.

Q: Do you think thirty thousand yen for each child afflicted was sufficient compensation in 1959?

HIGASHIDAIRA: Yes, certainly, given the value of that amount of money at the time. The families were very glad to get the money. Medical treatment didn't cost them anything, and it was the company that built the hospital in Minamata. We've done everything we can. If the victims hadn't been so poor, they probably would have gotten more money. In Japan, compensation is based on income. The Minamata fishers were barely able to earn enough to eat every day, and their prospects were quite limited. It's a mistake to compare payments made to them with those made to the victims of the gas explosion in Osaka [in 1970]. In that case, compensation of between twelve million and nineteen million yen was paid for young men at the peak of their powers. In Minamata the victims were almost all old people and children.

Q: For twenty-five years Chisso spent no money on treating its wastes. You must have channeled all the money you saved into production.

HIGASHIDAIRA: About fifty-fifty. The patients have cost us a considerable sum, you know.

Q: What do you think of the state of pollution in Japan?

HIGASHIDAIRA: The Japanese newspapers tend to make too much of a fuss over the issue. Let a feather drop onto their heads and they'll claim it was a whole bird. As for Minamata disease, that's an issue strictly between Chisso and the patients. It's a problem of the past and has nothing to do with current issues.

Q: What do you think of the trial?

HIGASHIDAIRA: Both the city and the prefecture oppose the trial. We've been forced into court. We'd prefer to resolve the problem out of court, in a friendly fashion, but they won't listen. Ninety percent of Minamata residents favor mediation. It's just a few who are creating a fuss. Only a hundred fifty people turn out for their demonstrations. Most citizens want to change the city's name. Some citizens even get together spontaneously and hold meetings in support of Chisso.

Q: I believe there's a growing antipollution movement in Minamata.

HIGASHIDAIRA: They're just trying to fan the hatred. Someone's out to agitate people. It wasn't so bad at first, but now it's become a witch hunt. The patients and their families come to us making demands, and sometimes a Buddhist priest stands outside the gate intoning a sutra of mourning. It's creepy.

Q: Would you feel the same about the way the company has handled the issue if your daughter had been one of the victims?

HIGASHIDAIRA: I can't even imagine that possibility.

Michiko could see that Chisso was quite unrepentant. She recalled the words of Hajime Hosokawa on his deathbed: "How are those children [congenital patients] doing? Oh, it's hard not to be able to help at such a critical time. There's no hope for Chisso. They should admit their responsibility."

Michiko had been visiting Hosokawa in the hospital. Gripping her hand in his, he had talked of Chisso's lack of moral responsibility and lamented the fate of the Minamata-disease patients. He died of lung cancer on October 13, 1970.

11. Smear Campaign

Kumamoto Prefecture's Pollution Victims Certification Board certified Teruo Kawamoto and seventeen others as Minamata-disease patients on October 6, 1971. This was done, however, only after Kawamoto had appealed to the Ministry of Health and Welfare to review the board's dubious certification procedures and the Environment Agency had censured the board.

Certification itself meant little to Kawamoto. He had fought long and hard despite his affliction. It was of little significance to him that he was now officially recognized to be suffering from Minamata disease. Certification did not alleviate his symptoms or protect him from discrimination and prejudice. Instead, he sought out fellow patients who had resigned themselves to suffering in silence and urged them to join him in his battle to force Chisso to accept responsibility for their plight.

No progress had been made in talks with Chisso since the heated give-and-take at the Mikasaya. On November 1, 1971, a newly formed group headed by Kawamoto demanded ¥30 million in compensation for each patient. Chisso turned the group down flat: "We will appeal to the Central Pollution Review Board [a commission established in the fall of 1970 as the successor to the Compensation Committee]. We refuse to pay even ¥10,000." Once again Chisso had passed the buck to a third party.

Angered, Kawamoto's group set up a tent in front of the entrance to Chisso's Minamata plant and settled in for a long siege. Recalling the humiliating defeat of the Mutual Aid Association back in 1959, Michiko feared that Kawamoto's group would not be able to stick together through a prolonged sit-in before Chisso's tightly shut gate. The group was backed by the Citizens' Council and the Association to Indict, but Michiko knew this was no guarantee that members of the group would not succumb to Chisso's promise of prompt payment if they agreed to the terms set by the Central Pollution Review Board. Already one family had given way to Chisso's pressure and agreed to accept a smaller payment.

As in 1959, there was little public support for the patients. In fact, the sit-in encouraged greater local support for Chisso. A fierce attack was launched on the patients through newspaper inserts accusing them of greed for demanding ¥30 million each in compensation. "Who do you think you are, a 'pollution elite'?" demanded one flier. "Destroy Chisso and you destroy Minamata."

Ever since Minamata disease had been officially labeled a pollution-related illness, Chisso had been hinting at withdrawing from Minamata. The company now intimated that compensation payments were proving too great a burden. One group of patients was demanding a total of ¥640 million, and now another group wanted ¥30 million a person. Minamata citizens had nightmares of Chisso staggering under the load and eventually abandoning the city. Fear of economic ruin fueled their hatred of the patients.

Newspaper inserts criticizing the patients began appearing almost daily; some days there were four or five. Their content grew more vicious by the day, innuendoes quickly escalating to direct attacks on the patients and their support groups.

Michiko could see that the newspaper inserts were fanning the same kind of hysteria that had erupted in 1959 and again in 1968. Chisso's tactics were effectively isolating the patients. But Michiko knew that the citizens' anger sprang from the city's dependence on Chisso. The citizens' subservience to Chisso was more to be pitied than censured.

The newspaper-insert smear campaign was triggered by two signature-collecting campaigns. One was led by a former Minamata deputy mayor, Katsuichi Watanabe, and a group he had formed called the Minamata Citizens' Council for Pollution Countermeasures. Watanabe had won a seat in the prefectural assembly with the support of Chisso's No. 2 Labor Union, which was loyal to management. His group, naturally, was fiercely protective of Chisso. The other campaign was conducted by a Liberal Democratic Party group led by Masahisa Tokutomi, head of the party's Minamata chapter; Misu Osaki, head of the chapter's women's division; and Koreharu Ogata, chairman of the Minamata Medical Association.

Both campaigns called upon national, prefectural, and municipal authorities to bring about an early resolution of the Minamata-disease issue. They urged that Minamata be cleansed of mercury and that the name of the disease be changed. There was no mention of Chisso's responsibility or the authorities' negligence. To Michiko and Kawamoto it was obvious that the campaigns were masterminded by Chisso. In protest they drew up a public appeal, which they distributed throughout the city on October 30. The text was Michiko's, a cry for the light of reason from the depths of oppressive darkness:

> To citizens of sound judgment: We newly certified patients have not been voluntarily afflicted with Minamata disease. Nor have we become sick simply to extract compensation from Chisso. We are sick because of the mercury-laden effluent Chisso has been pouring into the bay since 1932.
>
> Never will we forget the words of those who say, "You eat fish because you like it, so it's natural your arms and legs hurt. You've got money coming to you—why are you complaining?" When people plumb the depths, they can read the hearts and minds of others. After long years of struggle and pain, we have learned to read people's hearts.
>
> How can you expect those who live by the sea not to eat the fish they catch? What does it matter whether they like or

dislike fish? What else could they possibly have lived on all these years? And all the while they have hoped against hope that they would not be afflicted with that dreadful disease.

The first sign of disease in our own bodies and in the bodies of those close to us plunges us into an unimaginable hell. Not only is there the pain of illness; there is also the pain of prejudice and disdain. Why are we looked down upon? Why are we shunned? It is as if we had done something evil by becoming sick.

At the end of 1959, we were subjected to unspeakable humiliation, forced to accept the price of ¥300,000 for a life, ¥100,000 in place of good health, ¥30,000 for our children. We greeted the new year as cripples. Some of us went mad and died in mental hospitals; others were consigned to Minamata Municipal Hospital, where they died in agony cursing the Chisso disease, and then were cut up like fish on the Kumamoto University autopsy table. Still others, who should have been welcomed into the world with joy, were born with the disease.

We suffer from lack of work, lack of marriage partners, lack of friends. Still, we have fought to survive. One of us now in the hospital is receiving an annuity of ¥380,000 (the maximum paid so far). He would like to leave the hospital and live independently but, sadly, cannot survive without constant care. He is eligible for a nursing allowance of about ¥10,000 a month. But who is willing to care for someone for only ¥10,000, especially someone who has to live on ¥380,000 a year? Do you really think us lucky to get this money?

We newly certified patients had to put ourselves through the grinder, gaining certification only after appealing to the Ministry of Health and Welfare. Yet now that we have been certified, we find ourselves confronting the same loathing as in 1959, when the first patients received condolence payments; in 1968, when Minamata disease was finally recognized by the government as being caused by pollution; and in 1970, when the Compensation Committee issued its settlement proposal. We live in constant fear.

We ask those who are issuing the newspaper inserts against us to reply publicly to our appeal by November 3. Should there be no response, we will call on each and every one of you in person. We will do this fully aware of the inconvenience we cause you, for the sake of those of us who have suffered ignoble deaths and for the sake of our own souls.

More antipatient newspaper inserts with screaming headlines appeared: "What's Wrong with Cooperating with the Signature Campaigns? Are You Prepared to Take On the Whole City?" (November 6); "Explain Why You Need ¥30 Million!" (November 8); "Destroy the Company and What Is Left of Minamata?" (November 9). The campaign was escalating. One insert carried the transcript of what purported to be a dialogue among concerned Minamata citizens:

It is because the company is located in Minamata that express trains stop in this city of only fifty thousand people. Even the tourists come because the company is here. Company employees earn a lot of money, which they spend in Minamata. If the company left Minamata, every business in town would feel the effects. Consider what would happen to us then.

You who claim to have the support of the newly certified patients! You who would stir Minamata into a frenzy of confusion! Listen to the voices of Minamata's citizens! We recently held an open discussion among those who have cooperated with our signature campaigns. Listen to them, for they speak their true feelings. The participants desire to remain anonymous, so we have designated them A, B, C, and so on.

MODERATOR: You have played an active role in the signature-collecting campaigns. What views of the patients and their claims did people express to you?

A: Some said it was a pity the patients were being manipulated by a group of radicals just because people had been indifferent to them.

B: The people I talked to thought it was unfortunate that the rancor of a few unhappy employees in the company's No.

1 Labor Union coincided with the patients' greed. And since they chose the company as their target, they're having a hard time winning the sympathy of Minamata citizens.

c: What I heard was a lot harsher. "The patients are only thinking of themselves. They don't deserve any sympathy. And now [Katsuichi Watanabe's] campaign is promising them jobs and nursing care. This only encourages them. Ask them just how much it would take to satisfy them." I really didn't know how to reply.

d: One person really chewed me out. "The patients could be suffering from neuralgia or polio or maybe just alcoholism, but Katsuichi Watanabe is saying they should be given money and jobs and I don't know what all. I've already written directly to that idiot Teruo Kawamoto. I can't sign your petition, but I appreciate your hard work."

e: Everyone knows they got sick because they ate bad fish. The proof is that we've eaten just as much fish and we're not sick. No one who's bought fish from the local fish shops has gotten sick. Now, if they'd just eaten fish that had been caught and was being sold by *real* fishers . . .

MODERATOR: What do people think of the city councilwoman Fumiko Hiyoshi?

b: Some people said Hiyoshi seems to think all she has to do to get her way is cry. They said it was really something to see the way she could squeeze out those tears as if she were sick herself.

d: When a grown woman cries on TV, people who don't know her feel sorry for her. But those of us who know her just laugh and say, "Oh, is she at it again?"

c: The people I talked to wanted to know how a woman who had abandoned her own husband could feel love for anyone else. When she tries to drum up support for the patients, they think she's just trying to get publicity.

a: People told me Hiyoshi must think being on TV makes her a hero or something. . . . She probably plans to go on TV again at the next Chisso shareholders' meeting, since she owns a share.

D: Hiyoshi is a disgrace to Minamata. People are complaining that she's stirring up trouble not only here but in Tokyo and Osaka, too.

MODERATOR: The newly certified patients have been taking quite a high profile lately. How have people been reacting to them?

C: They're very unsympathetic. Kawamoto always used to come in first in the medical association's annual sports day, but he didn't even show up this year, I suppose because he was certified as a patient. People wonder if he's really sick.

B: Yes, a lot of people feel that way. Some even say there are people who faked their symptoms at the last group examination, practicing ahead of time so they wouldn't walk a straight line or show any reaction when they were pricked by a needle.

O: No one has anything good to say about their demand for thirty million yen, either. It's exorbitant, people are saying, much too much to get for simple neuralgia or alcoholism.

As you can see, the citizens of Minamata have no sympathy for you. Why do you suppose this is?

In your eagerness to bring down Chisso, in your greed for money, you have traveled around the country dressed like pilgrims and made a fuss at a Chisso shareholders' meeting, creating the impression that Minamata disease still exists. You must realize that your tactics have merely served to turn not only Chisso but also the citizens of Minamata against you. Your excessive demands are hurting other people.

Be warned: No matter who supports you, no matter what your reasons, *the citizens of Minamata will rise up as one to thwart your attempts to destroy Chisso.*

Allowing things to continue this way, Michiko saw, would only drive the patients into a corner from which they would never be able to extricate themselves. Help had to be sought outside Minamata's closed community. Keikichi Honda's arrival with reinforcements from Kumamoto City at this juncture was a godsend. On November 14 a rally was held in front of the

Chisso plant to show support for the eighteen families of Minamata-disease patients who were carrying on the sit-in there. Four busloads of Kumamoto University students swelled the crowd in front of the plant to more than five hundred.

Honda spoke first: "This sit-in is the start of a new battle in the war on Minamata disease. The first thing Chisso should do is seek out every patient living along the shores of the Shiranui Sea. Second, it should pay every one of these patients as much compensation as it can. We intend to persevere in this battle that the newly certified patients have launched."

He was followed by Fumiko Hiyoshi: "I have been called the disgrace of Minamata, but who is the real disgrace? Is it not those heartless Minamata citizens who are acting as Chisso's stooges in their attempts to destroy the patients? They say I cry too easily. But only a demon like Chisso could refrain from weeping at the sight of a congenital patient." The patients and their supporters then marched off under the wary eyes of riot police to weave their way through the streets of Minamata.

By uncanny coincidence, fifteen hundred people attended a citizens' rally at the municipal gymnasium the same day. Chisso executives, headed by the new president, Ken'ichi Shimada, were the guests of honor. The groups sponsoring the two signature-collecting campaigns merged at this rally to form the Citizens' Liaison Council for a Brighter Minamata. On his arrival in Minamata the day before, Shimada had announced that the company was donating ¥390 million for the construction of a culture center. He was welcomed at the rally by thunderous applause. "Minamata needs Chisso, after all," people murmured to one another.

The two rallies—one in support of the patients, the other in support of Chisso—symbolized the way in which Minamata had been split, or rather, the way in which a dedicated minority was being hounded by a larger, much more powerful group. As long as we stay here, thought Michiko, our feeble cries for ¥30 million are certain to be drowned out by Chisso's roar. We must go to Tokyo. In Tokyo we can appeal to a broader, disinterested public that will surely pronounce the kind of judgment upon Chisso that it deserves.

Michiko did not feel that the patients would make much headway pounding at the gate of Chisso's Minamata plant. Any demands they made would have to be referred to headquarters in any case. How could the patients' suffering be conveyed through so many intermediaries? We must go to Tokyo, she resolved, and confront Chisso management and the Chisso president. We must go to Tokyo, as we did once before.

Kawamoto, leader of the patients' group, agreed. Now that the patients had compelled the government authorities to recognize their condition, they should not wait for a court verdict but should boldly confront the Chisso leadership, negotiating directly with the president and forcing the company to make restitution. "Michiko," he said, "let's go to Tokyo as soon as possible." For Kawamoto and the families of the newly certified Minamata patients, the road to Tokyo was the road to regeneration and the reinstatement of their humanity. Unlike the patients who had taken their case to court, this group had chosen to fight Chisso directly, without government intervention.

Michiko could tell that Kawamoto was fully aware of the struggle ahead. "It will be hard, but yes, let's go," she replied. In 1970, she had gone to Tokyo to take part in the May 25 action to protest the Compensation Committee's proposed settlement, and had also been present at the inauguration of the Tokyo chapter of the Association to Indict. This trip, she knew, would be different. The Kumamoto trial was still in progress. Michiko would have to travel constantly between Kumamoto City and Tokyo if she were to continue her support for the patients fighting in court and at the same time help the new group of patients take on Chisso directly. This group was in for a grim battle with no end in sight.

The patients and their supporters would need money. Where was it to come from? There was the Paradise of the Bitter Sea Fund, supported by contributions from sympathizers throughout Japan, but it was barely adequate to alleviate the financial burden of individual patients. It could not underwrite an extended confrontation with Chisso. The circle of support would have to be enlarged. It would be necessary to solicit donations from passersby in the streets of Tokyo and to ask writers and other intellectuals she knew for support.

Michiko's mother and husband encouraged her, but the citizens of Minamata were not so understanding. "She's certain to make better money in the big city," they said sarcastically. "After all, she's become famous thanks to Minamata disease."

Before Michiko left for Tokyo, she wanted to say goodbye to terminally ill friends. One was Masae Fuchigami, who had a fourteen-year-old daughter born with the disease. Fuchigami had belonged to the group of patients in favor of taking Chisso to court, but life had become too difficult and she had dropped out, accepting a lump-sum payment from Chisso. She had just built a new house. She had once been renowned in the area for her beauty, but now her face was wasted by illness.

"I can't die first, Michiko. I'd have to kill this child before I could die."

"You've just built a wonderful house," said Michiko, trying to cheer her. "You have to hurry up and get well so you can enjoy it." She knew, though, that her words had little meaning to one who was dying.

"Oh, Michiko, I'll soon be going to a place where I won't need a house. I won't need anything." Smiling sadly, Fuchigami feebly squeezed Michiko's hand. And so the two women parted, one bound for death, the other for a battle to the death.

12. Confrontation in Tokyo

ON DECEMBER 7, 1971, Kawamoto met Shimada for the first time. Visiting him at Chisso's Tokyo headquarters, Kawamoto handed over his group's list of demands and requested that Chisso reply the next day.

On December 8 two hundred supporters, including members of the Association to Indict, stood guard outside the fourth-floor conference room where Kawamoto's group was meeting with Shimada. Every one of the supporters wore on his or her breast a black square of cloth bearing the words "Minamata *shimin*," or "the Minamata dead," in white. (This was an ironic play on words: *shimin*, meaning "citizen," was written with characters pronounced the same way but bearing the very different meaning of "dead person.") The idea had been Michiko's, a fitting symbol, she thought, of the retribution they sought for the many who had died of Minamata disease.

Chisso was taken aback by the unexpected appearance of the supporters. Fearing for their president's safety, a number of executives tried to force their way through the crowd to the conference room but were thwarted by the "Minamata dead." Not even orders from Mitsubishi Estate Company, which managed the building, to leave the premises immediately could move the supporters. Irritated Chisso employees began yelling at the supporters: "Get out, you're in the way, we can't work!"

"Work?" came the reply. "Who robbed us of our work and our lives?"

Plainclothes police soon appeared, ostensibly to investigate the possibility that Chisso's president was being held against his will, but left after witnessing the give-and-take between the patients and Shimada. The electric atmosphere in the room precluded interference.

While Michiko and the others in the room watched with bated breath, Kawamoto took out a razor and stepped up to Shimada. "We want your word written in blood. Come on, all you have to do is cut your finger. Can't you do that, Mr. President? Can't you understand the patients' pain? Don't you feel their suffering?" Tears streaming down his cheeks, Kawamoto shook Shimada by the lapels. Shimada's face was ashen.

"I can't do that. Please understand. I can't do that."

"I'm not telling you to cut off your finger. Just a little nick. Come on, come on. Cut it, cut it."

"Please . . ."

For more than a decade Chisso's president—Kiichi Yoshioka, Yutaka Egashira, and now Ken'ichi Shimada—had turned a deaf ear to the patients' demands. Now Shimada seemed at a loss for words. It was both a dramatic and a pathetic sight. Michiko stood quietly in a corner, watching the confrontation. Kawamoto made no attempt to wipe away his tears; he seemed possessed by the anguished spirits of the dead patients.

KAWAMOTO: I've come to set the record straight once and for all. I've come today determined to get our demands written in blood. We'll write them together, you and I.

SHIMADA: What?

KAWAMOTO: We're going to write them in blood. Come on, cut my finger.

SHIMADA: Please, I can't.

KAWAMOTO: I'll cut your finger. We'll do it together.

SHIMADA: Please, please.

KAWAMOTO: If you won't do it, I'll have to do it alone. I'll cut my own finger. I've come prepared. "Please, please," you say. There's no "please" about it. Come on, cut my finger and I'll write. And I'll cut your finger and you'll write. We'll both hurt.

That's fair, isn't it? You're human, why can't we share the same pain?

SHIMADA: Please, I can't do that.

KAWAMOTO: Here you are, here you are. Come on, cut, cut, cut. I'm not leaving until you do. I didn't come all the way to Tokyo just for show. We're still holding our own back in Minamata. We've still got our tent up in front of your factory. There are old men there. It's hard on them, but they're sticking it out. Can you understand how hard it is for them? Can you? Come on, cut, cut, cut. Let's suffer this together.

SHIMADA: Please, I can't do that.

KAWAMOTO: We'll both write [the demands]. Here, cut. Cut, I say. We've got to write them today. We've been entrusted with this mission.

SHIMADA: No, I can't do that.

KAWAMOTO: Now, now. We're both human. We can suffer this together. You can do that much.

SHIMADA: Please, forgive me.

KAWAMOTO: There's no "forgive me" about it. I'm not giving up. Not today, not ever. You may be laughing inside, but we don't have time for laughter. We've got to go back to Minamata. There are still a hundred sixty patients who've applied for certification, and they haven't even been examined yet. There may be thousands more. Come on, now, Mr. President, cut, I say. If you don't, I will. And I'll cut your finger, too.

SHIMADA: Please, Mr. Kawamoto. Don't cut your finger.

KAWAMOTO: I will, I will. We used all our resources to come to Tokyo. We spent money scraped together from donations from all over the country to come here.

NOBUO MIYAZAWA: You people think this issue can be judged by how serious the disease is. Han'naga was certified in April, but he's been sick since 1946. Where did you rank him, eh? How much did you decide he was worth?

SHIMADA: I'm sorry, I don't remember.

MIYAZAWA: That's all our suffering is to you. I'll tell you. Han'naga got an annuity of two hundred ninety thousand yen. He has a child born with Minamata disease, you know. His wife has left him. He lives with his old mother. How does that kind of suffering work out to two hundred ninety thousand yen? Explain that. [Shimada remains silent.] We put the same question to Kuga and Higashidaira. They just told us the Compensation Committee had decided on the amount and that both sides had agreed to it. Now you're trying to do the same thing.

MASARU ISHIDA [shaking spasmodically]: Can you really understand the patients' pain? You can stick needles into my child and he doesn't feel a thing. He was born with Minamata disease. Do you have any idea what that's like?

KAWAMOTO [sobbing]: If you can share our pain, cut my finger. If you can understand my pain, cut. I didn't come all the way to Tokyo just for show.

[One by one, the patients cut their fingers. They close in on Shimada. Their blood drips onto the tabletop. Someone tries to write the characters for *petition* on the paper they have brought, but the blood smears and the word is barely legible.]

SHIMADA: Please, not that.

MICHIKO: The patients never had a chance to say, "Please, not that," when they were stricken with Minamata disease. What could they have wanted less?

KANJI IRIE [a Chisso director]: Wait a minute. Let me talk to Mr. Shimada.

KAWAMOTO: Shut up. What could you have to talk to him about?

IRIE: Just for a moment.

KAWAMOTO: We won't be fooled. Come on, give me your finger.

SHIMADA: Please.

KAWAMOTO: Please, please, please. I'm the one who's saying please. I'm the one who's saying, "Please, not that." [He sobs.]

IRIE: Just for a moment. I've got something to say to Mr. Shimada.

KAWAMOTO: What are you going to do with these people? Takeharu Sato, here, his wife hasn't been able to function as a wife or mother for more than ten years. And you talk about "questionable" patients and "authentic" patients. Who do you think you are?

ISHIDA: You came and saw for yourself, didn't you? You saw my child. You saw Sato's wife. But you still don't understand.

KAWAMOTO: No one on the Central Pollution Review Board is going to understand. They know nothing about Minamata disease.

ISHIDA: All you give us are words. People like you can't possibly understand our pain.

[The confrontation continues far into the night, but no progress is made. Finally Shimada collapses from hypertension. The patients slump to the floor in exhaustion.]

KAWAMOTO: I'm all feverish. I can't think straight anymore. It's sad to have to confront a sick man like this.

IRIE: I understand.

KAWAMOTO: Our behavior must shock you. It must seem awful, the way we're badgering this sick man.

IRIE: I haven't said that. It's just that we've got this situation here. Don't worry; we will definitely respond to your petition.

KAWAMOTO [sobbing]: Oh, we haven't gotten anywhere.

IRIE: Please, Mr. Kawamoto, don't cry like that.

TAKEHARU SATO: It would be one thing if you were prepared to take responsibility, but you're just running away from it, aren't you?

IRIE: I'm not running away.

KAWAMOTO: So we come out looking like villains.

SATO: If you were sincere, you'd accept responsibility, since your president is indisposed. You'd take over, since he can't continue.

IRIE: But this is a very important issue. Only the president can resolve it.

SATO: Well, if you won't take responsibility, who will? Where does that leave us?

IRIE: That's why I'm saying let him go for now.

KAWAMOTO: Go ahead, leave. Go on. We're not getting anywhere, anyway.

IRIE: Mr. Kawamoto, please stop crying. I understand.

KAWAMOTO: Why do we have to try so hard? Go on, leave. Go on.

IRIE: He'll give you an answer later. Just let him rest a while.

KAWAMOTO: I don't even want to see him anymore. Go on, leave.

MICHIKO [speaking softly, kindly]: Mr. Irie, when did you ever call a doctor for a Minamata-disease patient who had come to see you?

KAWAMOTO: Never mind, never mind. Go on, leave, leave. I don't care what happens now. We've been at it for twelve hours, thirteen hours, and look where we are. Go on, leave, I say. Leave.

SATO: Hurry up, take him [Shimada] with you.

IRIE: Please just wait a bit for our response.

[They begin to move the stretcher bearing Shimada. Kawamoto crawls toward the stretcher, sobbing.]

KAWAMOTO: Do you know why I'm crying? My father slept all alone. I fed him three times a day. We had so little to eat. I pawned my suits, everything. What can you know about a life like that? There were so many times we had no food for the next day. We didn't even have bedding, and it was always so cold, so cold. What do you know about such suffering? We were almost thrown out of our own home, you know. Is thirty million yen really so much? My father died at sixty-nine. I cried when he died. He died in a psychiatric hospital, in a room like a prison cell, all alone. What can you know about such pain? Have you ever been to a psychiatric hospital? He died in a lousy psychiatric hospital, locked in a room all by himself. I've never told anyone about this before. I know something about nursing; I can tell you're really sick. I know what a heart attack is like. I know about high blood pressure.

After thirteen hours, Chisso's president was carried out of the room on a stretcher. It was late at night. Kawamoto clung to the stretcher.

There was no one left with whom to negotiate. After a quick conference, the patients decided to remain where they were until they received a sincere response to their demands. That night they slept on the cold floor outside the president's office. Someone had brought in blankets. Michiko slept with the patients, wrapping herself in a blanket against the December chill.

When she closed her eyes, she saw the Shiranui Sea glittering, and far off the golden hills of the Amakusa Islands. The cape is bursting with flowers: camellias, milk vetch, tangerine blossoms. Mayflies dance amid the fragrant profusion. The small inlet is smooth as a mirror. Only the white wake of a passing boat disturbs its calm, gentle ripples, which spread until they touch the deep green shore. The cape's reflection in the water undulates slightly. A man waves from a small fishing boat. It is Susumu Sugimoto. Has he had a good catch today, perhaps? There is his beloved daughter, Eiko, laughing. Children run along the beach, calling out in welcome.

Soon the blue inlet is wrapped in a gray mist. Sugimoto's sad face looms in the mist. "I'd like to go out just once more," he says. A fishing boat rests on the shore, mired in mercury-impregnated sludge. Michiko hears the voice of Yuki Sakagami: "In the evenings I think about the sea more than anything. It was good being on the sea. . . . I want to use my own arms and legs to go rowing out after *aosa* just one more time. I want to go so bad I could cry. Just one more time."

The leaden mist disappears, and once again the Shiranui Sea is a glittering blue. The image fades.

In the middle of the night on December 24, the seventeenth day of their sit-in at Chisso's Tokyo headquarters, Michiko and the patients found themselves thrown out onto the cold sidewalk. Tokyo was in a festive mood, for it was Christmas Eve. That day Michiko, Kawamoto, and Sato had been warming themselves around a makeshift *kotatsu,* a low, quilt-covered table with a heater under it. Throughout the sit-in, Michiko and Kawamoto had been fasting in protest. They were exhausted and were resting their heads on the table. Suddenly a number of Chisso executives appeared with a message from Shimada. The group included Kuga, now a director; Tsuchiya, now director of general affairs; and Tsuneya Kawashima, director of personnel.

The talks had been suspended on the pretext of Shimada's sudden illness. He now promised to resume negotiations in Minamata as soon as he had recovered, and asked the patients and their supporters to leave the building. When they refused, a contingent of Chisso employees elbowed their way into the conference room and dragged twenty supporters into the corridor, then dragged others out of the reception room. Finally only Michiko, Kawamoto, and Sato remained, seated in front of the president's office.

Kuga squatted down before Kawamoto. "Look, the Central Pollution Review Board isn't going to change its mind, no matter what. There's no point pressing for talks here. Go back to Minamata. Shimada will go there eventually to work out something with you."

What was the point of returning to Minamata? Kawamoto protested. Hadn't they come all the way to Tokyo precisely because they weren't getting anywhere in Minamata? The patients sitting patiently in front of the Chisso plant in Minamata had pinned their hopes on the talks at Chisso headquarters in Tokyo. They simply couldn't go back to those people empty handed.

Kuga tried first cajolery, then threats, but nothing could budge Kawamoto. Kuga took out an envelope of money and threw it on the table. "If you won't go home, let's go to an inn or a hotel to talk."

Kawamoto crossed his arms and tilted backward until he was lying flat on the floor looking up at the ceiling. His lips remained tightly closed.

"All right, all right. I give up." Tucking the envelope back into his pocket, Kuga marched off in a huff.

This blatant attempt at bribery disgusted Michiko. Kawamoto and Sato were equally taken aback. Money must have been Chisso's tactic in getting the Minamata Fishermen's Cooperative on its side, Michiko thought.

Suddenly the door swung open to reveal a crowd of Chisso employees.

"We want you to leave."

The three found themselves surrounded.

"We won't leave of our own volition." Kawamoto and Sato sat rigidly, their arms crossed.

Hands shot out, and the two were carried off kicking and squirming in protest. Michiko turned to gather their belongings.

"You, too." Her arms were gripped tightly as she was hustled out of the room. Where had the other two been taken? Where would she be taken? Michiko felt helpless. How pitiful she must look, she thought. After turning numerous corners along a dark corridor, Michiko found herself thrown outside.

Patients and supporters came running up to her. "Are you all right? Kawamoto and Sato are fine. We were worried about you." The words were spoken in relief, but Michiko's mind was in turmoil. Where could they possibly go now? They had to find a place to stay. Where would they get the money? They would need pots and pans to cook with, dishes and cups, bedding and heating to survive the cold.

The students who had come to support their cause had set up a tent in front of the building, and it was decided that they would stay there. The tent was warm with the affection and support of the young students.

Outraged by Chisso's rough treatment of Michiko and the patients, a group of thirty-three intellectuals signed a letter of protest to Chisso, which was delivered by thirteen members of the group and a number of supporters on December 29. That day the patients, accompanied by Michiko and Keikichi Honda, had gone again to Chisso headquarters. They were followed by the thirteen intellectuals, led by Genzaburo Yoshino, a commentator; Rokuro Hidaka, a sociologist; Yoko Matsuoka, a commentator; Yuko Mochizuki, a Diet member; Ken'ichi Tanigawa, a commentator; and Hidenobu Ueno, a writer. The Chisso security guards were ready and waiting, and the group had to force its way to the designated meeting place, the area in front of the elevator on the fourth floor. Several supporters were injured in the fray, but finally everyone made it to the meeting place.

The patients lost no time in once again presenting their case to Chisso. They would settle for nothing less than direct negotiations with Shimada, they said, but Kuga and the other Chisso executives would have none of it. The president was too ill, they declared. The only avenue of protest they would recognize was the Central Pollution Review Board. After much shouting back and forth, Yoshino, who had come despite his age and frailty, began reading aloud the letter of protest. The meeting place subsided into silence as the old liberal's dignified voice rang out:

> What kind of conduct is it to refuse to respond to the patients, who have come all the way to Tokyo as a last resort? What kind of conduct is it to ignore them totally and then throw them out into the street? They came in good faith. Your attitude can only be termed inhuman. As people who have taken part in the sit-in or wish we could have, we must protest the recent events.
>
> Why do you refuse to comply with the request of the patients and their families for direct, unconditional negotiations? Why do you remain adamant, even resorting to violence?
>
> We believe that no more time should be lost. Chisso and the patients should meet directly to discuss compensation arrangements that will be satisfactory to both sides. This would be the first step toward making restitution to the many who have been killed or crippled, to the many who have been made to suffer pain they never deserved.
>
> It need hardly be said that direct negotiations are only the first small step toward a final resolution. We will maintain a vigilant watch over the progress that is made.

Not content with this, Ueno and another member of the group, Nao'o Harada, editor of the magazine *Tembo,* began a hunger strike in front of Chisso headquarters on New Year's Eve to protest the prejudice and violence visited on the patients. They continued their hunger strike through the first three days of 1972. The patients, too, welcomed the new year still ensconced in the tent outside Chisso headquarters. They could hear the year being ushered in by the whistles of the ships moored at nearby Harumi pier.

This year did not promise to be any easier than the last, but Michiko resolved anew to persevere in the battle for direct negotiations, no matter how long and bitter the struggle.

Sad news arrived early in January: Masae Fuchigami, whom Michiko had visited just before leaving Minamata for Tokyo, had died on January 4. A new soul had come to rest on Michiko's shoulders. She had left behind a daughter severely afflicted with the disease and totally helpless. There could be no rest for Michiko's weary soul until the patients won their fight for direct negotiations.

Whenever one of their companions died, the patients were plunged into despair. They too had been poisoned by mercury; they too would soon become sad spirits. Their fight was a fight against death itself; how much harder it was to wage battle so far from home. Michiko's constant presence and kind attention were their sole consolation. She had shared everything with them: the trip up from Minamata, the sit-in, the siege of Chisso headquarters, the petitioning for monetary contributions, the hunger strike. However depressed they were, the patients could be revived by a word of encouragement from Michiko.

The support of the group of Tokyo intellectuals also encouraged the patients. The letter of protest that Yoshino had read epitomized the patients' anger, stifled for so many years. Michiko's *Paradise of the Bitter Sea* had won formidable allies.

People stopped by the tent, leaving gifts and money to express their support and offering words of encouragement. Such gestures of public support were another source of comfort to the patients, the goodwill of strangers brightening, if only briefly, their bleak lives. They knew that they owed this kindness to Michiko, too, for it was her deft portrayal of the patients as victims that had attracted so much sympathy. Every day the sit-in continued, Chisso's image as an inhuman entity was engraved deeper and deeper into the consciousness of Tokyo citizens.

Why, thought Michiko in anger, did Chisso insist on physically obstructing every attempt of the patients to enter into direct negotiations? The company had created a security force that threw out any patients or supporters who tried to enter the building. Most members of this force, it was later learned, were workers from Chisso's plant in Goi, Chiba Prefecture. After consulting with Michiko, Kawamoto decided to deliver a petition to Hideo Natsume, head of the Federation of Chisso Labor Unions, who was working at the Goi plant, asking what the true intent behind the company's attempts to obstruct negotiations was and requesting that union members refrain from interfering with negotiations.

Natsume agreed over the phone to receive the petition from Kawamoto at 11:00 A.M. on January 7. Early that morning Kawamoto boarded the train for Goi, petition in hand. He was accompanied by four companions and a contingent of journalists. No one thought the meeting would go smoothly. Indeed, there might be no discussion at all; handing over the petition might be all that Kawamoto could do. Sure enough, when he arrived at the Chisso plant, he found the factory gate closed and a number of tight-faced guards standing watch. When Kawamoto stated that he had an appointment with Natsume, he was told, "Natsume has to consult with the federation. He doesn't have the authority to agree on his own to meet with you."

After two hours in the bitter cold, Kawamoto gave up. "Could you at least give this petition to Mr. Natsume?" he asked the guards.

"You'll have to hand it to him personally. We can't take it for you," was the response.

Disgusted, one of the reporters vaulted the gate. The gate opened, and after a moment's hesitation those waiting outside moved through. Further obstacles awaited them, however. They were told Natsume had gone to Tokyo for a meeting at Chisso headquarters and could not contact them until 3:00 P.M. Kawamoto was too tired to argue. He asked if he could rest inside the gatehouse. Around two hundred men suddenly appeared.

"Attack!"

The men fell upon the group. They did not seem to care whether they attacked patients or reporters.

"Hey, this one's a patient!"

"Who gives a damn!"

Kawamoto, who was wearing a white sash bearing the words "Minamata-disease patient," was shoved around and kicked in the face. He was covered with blood. Among the photographers present was Eugene Smith, accompanied by his wife, Aileen. He was dragged outside the gate, punched in the face and stomach, and pushed to the ground. He covered his eyes and lost consciousness. Someone dragged Aileen down by the hair. Cries pierced the air. Groans of pain could be heard everywhere. No one was spared—not the patients, not their supporters, not the reporters and photographers. The Chisso thugs did their job well. Hurling insults, they vanished.

Chisso's vicious attack on the patients stirred a public outcry. The day after the Goi incident, one thousand people gathered in a hall in Tokyo to protest Chisso's extreme tactics. A shaken Kawamoto reported what had happened. "At the order to attack they fell upon us. We were dragged down and stepped on. This is Chisso's real face. But we won't give up. We'll continue our sit-in in Tokyo even if it means becoming beggars. I ask your continued support." The audience burst into applause.

After this, Michiko introduced the patients. She had had a cold since December 8, yet she had participated in the hunger strike and had joined the patients in their sit-in outside Chisso headquarters. She appeared worn and fragile. But there was strength in the hand clutching the microphone, which she extended to the patients as she introduced them.

"I want to fight, not just as a patient but as a human being," said Takeharu Sato. By him sat his wheelchair-bound wife, Yae, who had just arrived in Tokyo to encourage her husband in his battle. Since she could not sit comfortably for long in the wheelchair, Takeharu carried her to the stage and laid her down. Haltingly, she spoke: "I don't know how to thank you for coming here. There are so many of you. Perhaps the past eighteen years of suffering have not been for nothing. I would like for a day, or even just an hour, to be able to walk like you and work like you." There was no sound from the audience.

"We may be forsaken by some, but there are also those who wish to help us," said Michiko. "There is a sweet-potato vender who comes to our tent in front of Chisso headquarters to give us hot baked sweet potatoes. There are those who bring money they have collected at their New Year's parties. There appears to be no end to your warm sympathy and support. You give us the courage to continue our battle."

The meeting broke up, to convene again outside for a protest march. Led by Yae Sato in her wheelchair, the mass of people flowed toward the center of the city, black banners bearing the white character *on* (rancor) fluttering above their heads.

13. THE BELEAGUERED GIANT

IT WAS JANUARY 11, 1972. Michiko and the patients had arrived at Chisso headquarters to make their usual protest. Michiko drew in her breath sharply upon stepping out of the elevator on the building's fourth floor. The next instant everyone burst out laughing. The entryway to all the floor's rooms had been blocked off with a row of steel bars. Having failed to discourage the patients through violence, Chisso had apparently decided to lock itself behind bars. The sight was both comical and sad.

"Just like a zoo! But Chisso is, after all, an economic animal," joked the patients as they ran their hands over the thick bars.

Lifting a megaphone to his mouth, Kawamoto called out to the people on the other side of the bars, "You have erected a truly historic monument. Do you really think these bars are going to keep us out?"

The press was delighted with the bars, and photos of the barricaded fourth floor appeared in the newspapers. Sightseers poured in daily to view the barricade. After gazing at the sight, they apparently felt compelled to say something to the people on the other side, for they would invariably hurl an insult before leaving.

The bars were obviously meant to keep the patients out, but to Michiko they seemed to lock in the very people who had put them up. Chisso was caught in its own trap; the bars only made people more curious and exposed Chisso's shame to the public.

On January 24 a Buddhist memorial service for the Minamata dead was held before the bars. The names of the dead were written above an altar bearing their memorial tablets and photographs. Incense wafted through the bars, and the rhythmic drone of chanted sutras echoed through the building.

When the sutra chanting was finished, Michiko stepped up to the altar to speak. "It is with fond recollection that we remember you in life. All is like a fading dream. I cast myself before you not because of anything you said or did but because of my deep sorrow. All worldly ties are like wraiths in the darkness." Her voice rang out strong and true, stopping people in their tracks and guiding them to Chisso's fourth floor.

According to the old lunar calendar, February 4 is the day before spring. On this day it is traditional to scatter parched beans around the house, chanting, "Demons out, fortune in!" That day Michiko and the patients threw beans between the steel bars, shouting, "Demons in, fortune out! Demons in, fortune out!" The patients had been pinned in a corner by Chisso for so long. It was high time their roles were reversed, if only for a brief, exhilarating moment. Michiko could not help smiling to herself, the patients were enjoying themselves so thoroughly.

The steel barricade provided the patients with a physical entity against which to vent their rage, but it also cut off all possibility of direct negotiations with Chisso. Once again driven to action by Chisso's underhanded tactics, on February 10 Nao'o Harada and the other intellectuals who supported the patients appealed to the Central Pollution Review Board to turn down Chisso's request for the board's arbitration and thus clear the way for direct negotiations between the company and Kawamoto's group.

The director general of the Environment Agency, Buichi Oishi, also began to press Chisso to give up its attempt to hide behind the board. This apparently had an effect, for on February 14 Chisso withdrew its request for arbitration. The patients had won the fight for direct negotiations.

Once the two sides were talking again, the patients indicated their willingness to negotiate for less than the ¥30 million per patient they had originally demanded. As long as Chisso showed a sincere desire to do something for them, they said, they were prepared to settle for an amount closer to that being demanded by the patients who had chosen to take the matter to court, and they presented the figure of ¥18 million per patient. This did not mean, however, that the patients' bitterness had faded. "Money can't compensate us for the grief we have to bear. At least we should be allowed to set the price, since we're the only ones who know how much we suffer," they muttered. When negotiations were officially resumed on April 21, the patients could not resist voicing their deeply rooted dissatisfaction.

"We're settling for eighteen million yen only because we want to be sure to get something. You can't wipe out our pain or our families' pain, no matter how much you pay us. It's not as if we're going to get any better. It's not as if we're going to stop suffering prejudice and discrimination."

"Of course we don't think money is going to relieve you of your suffering. But as a company, the only way we can do anything to compensate is to give you money."

"If you really felt sorry, you'd show us everything you've got and tell us to take whatever we wanted. You can't trade a person's life and health for any amount of cash. You should be willing to pay us all you've got to show that you realize this. As it is, we're not asking much. No, a hundred million yen, two hundred million yen, wouldn't be enough. Only the person who's suffering can put a price tag on that suffering. You ought to realize that."

"There's just no way to compensate you except with money. It has nothing to do with how much a life is worth."

"This is a basic human problem. Because of your mercury, innocent people have been hurt. I didn't become a cripple because you and I physically fought each other. People were living peacefully, and suddenly they were hurt for no reason. All so you could make a profit."

The talks continued in this vein. Michiko could see that the Chisso people still could not comprehend the absolute value of human life. The patients' pleas were falling on deaf ears. Deep within her was an emptiness that ached with the patients' pain.

Among those present was Issei Sawada, who had recently succeeded Kosaku Teramoto as governor of Kumamoto Prefecture. After a while he stood up. "You're talking at cross-purposes. We're not going to get anywhere this way. I declare the talks ended for today." He was followed out of the conference room by the greatly relieved Chisso representatives. The patients were left alone.

Later that year, Chisso employees filed charges against Kawamoto, accusing him of having assaulted and injured them at Chisso's Tokyo headquarters. On October 30 the police took him in for questioning. One of those filing charges was a worker who had been transferred from the Goi plant to guard the steel barricade in Tokyo. Another was Tsuneya Kawashima, Chisso's personnel director, who headed the so-called defense force and who was rumored to have used violence against the patients and their supporters many times himself. Chisso had photographs taken during some of the more heated confrontations with the patients, which, it was claimed, proved Chisso's case.

Michiko was disgusted by Chisso's tactics. After repeated efforts to coerce the patients and after physically harming them, Chisso had the gall to turn the tables and claim to be the victim, all on the basis of a handful of photographs that showed little more than a patient grabbing someone's sleeve in the heat of argument. How typical of Chisso, thought Michiko. It had been like this ever since Minamata disease had become an issue.

And what about the police? Chisso was accused of mass poisoning, but the company had never been investigated by the police. Yet when the patients created a fuss, the police were right there to apply pressure. It was just like 1959, when the fishers had fought their fiercest fight against Chisso. The police had stood by until the fishers had been backed so far into a corner that they lashed out in anger. Then, and only then, did the police move in to arrest the fishers at Chisso's instigation. As far as Michiko and the patients were concerned, Chisso and the police were in collusion.

The Metropolitan Police Department's Public Security Division dispatched detectives to search the dormitory in which the patients and some supporters were staying and even had thirteen detectives travel all the way to Minamata to search Kawamoto's house. When he reported voluntarily to the Marunouchi police station, an officer hinted darkly of imminent arrest and yelled, "Don't get cocky just because you're a pollution patient!" (He was interrogated not by Marunouchi police but by officers of a special division set up to investigate ultraleftist violence.)

Throughout the struggle to bring Chisso to the negotiating table, the patients had never filed criminal charges against anyone working for the company: not when Chisso workers beat them, not when blood was streaming down their faces, not even when their bones were broken.

"If we charge Chisso with inflicting injury on us when it's responsible for a much graver crime, we'll only obscure our real suffering," Michiko had argued. Yet here was Chisso trying to divert attention from its own crime by accusing the victims of that crime of inflicting scratches on its employees.

Only Michiko and a few younger women were present the day the police came to search the patients' dormitory. Michiko was also staying there at the time, commuting to Chisso headquarters daily to take part in the sit-in and, whenever she could find time, working on *Ten no Uo* (Fish of Heaven), the second sequel to *Paradise of the Bitter Sea*, which was appearing in serial form in the magazine *Tembo*, in order to raise badly needed funds. (The first sequel had been serialized in the monthly magazine *Henkyo* in 1970 and 1971 but had been left unfinished.)

Fatigue had ruined Michiko's eyesight. She had just had the lens of her left eye removed. Her right eye had also weakened greatly, and she had to use a magnifying glass to read. She was still recovering from the operation when the police arrived, and could not read the search warrant that was thrust before her. She had the police read the warrant out loud so that she could record it on tape.

Kawamoto had left that morning to report to the Maruno-uchi police station. The other patients had accompanied him, while most of the young supporters staying in the dormitory had left as usual for the tent pitched outside Chisso headquarters.

The young women were flustered by the sudden invasion. "Stop squawking and act your age," yelled a policeman.

"Please speak more politely," said Michiko crisply. She continued, "I don't know what you're searching for, but please handle things carefully. Everything here has been donated to the patients by citizens of this city."

As she spoke, one of the policemen held up the splint Kawamoto had been using after having broken a toe at Chisso's Tokyo headquarters. Flakes of plaster broke off as the police busily took its measurements. "We'll take this, if you don't mind," one of them said. Kawashima, a fifth-*dan* judo wrestler, had charged that Kawamoto, who was considerably smaller, had assaulted him with the splint. Surely, thought Michiko, the police knew that Kawamoto had required the splint in the first place because he had been hurt by Chisso employees.

After the police had left, Michiko went with Rokuro Hidaka and another member of the support group of intellectuals, the commentator Kunio Maruyama, to the Marunouchi police station to protest Kawamoto's being taken in for questioning. They presented a statement of protest signed by ninety-three supporters. "How can you dare to hinder the patients' efforts to crawl out from under the unimaginable oppression they suffer?" the statement asked, and went on to criticize the extraordinary zeal with which the police were investigating the charges against the patients instead of trying to help them.

The protest was to no avail. On December 27 Kawamoto was indicted.

"Michiko, an awful thing has happened," said Kawamoto. He proceeded to tell her about the use of forged documents to manipulate some of the patients. As she listened to his tale, Michiko was shocked once again at the lengths to which those in power would go to sweep the weak out of their way.

The issue revolved around the growing number of patients being certified as suffering from Minamata disease. In January 1973, two months before the verdict in the Kumamoto trial was due, the Central Pollution Review Board was renamed the Environmental Dispute Coordination Commission and invested with more-binding powers. This body immediately began working out a proposal for compensation payments to the patients Chisso had persuaded to accept a mediated settlement, in the hope of undercutting the amounts the court was thought likely to award.

On January 10 it was revealed that the request for mediation and the document of power of attorney that had supposedly been presented to the commission by the patients were forgeries. The patients did not recall giving anyone such sweeping powers to represent them and claimed that they had never even seen the documents. Kawamoto, who had been meeting with the patients who had chosen to accept the commission's decision, had become suspicious. That day, accompanied by a number of other patients and members of the press, he went to the commission and demanded to be shown the documents in question. After several hours, during which the commission members tried to deny him this right, it was revealed to one and all that some of the patients' signatures and seals had been forged. The newspapers lost no time in reporting the incident.

It turned out that the documents had been prepared by employees of the Minamata city office's Pollution Division. The patients' anger toward Chisso blazed anew. One after another, they withdrew their requests for mediation.

The Environmental Dispute Coordination Commission and Minamata City—and, by extension, Chisso—had hoped to take advantage of the patients' unfamiliarity with legal procedures and their willingness to trust others. "The Minamata city employees acted in good faith, thinking they were helping the patients" was Chisso's lame excuse for the fraud.

Not even the commission could withstand the criticism of the press and the general public. The chairman of the commission was replaced, and the new chairman promised to follow due process and to refrain from reaching a settlement until the Kumamoto trial was concluded. The patients had managed to foil this crude attempt to influence the judge's decision on compensation by cobbling together a settlement that would award patients only minimal compensation.

Michiko knew better than anyone else how close the patients had come to being swindled. The government commission had been appalled at the rapidly growing number of certified patients. There were those in positions of power who feared that the Minamata issue would trigger a nationwide antipollution movement. The sooner the embarrassment of Minamata disease could be forgotten, the better. Accomplishing this necessitated dividing the patients, thus confusing the issue so that the general public would quickly lose interest. The commission was only a tool being manipulated to that end.

Never would Michiko forget how the Compensation Committee had attempted similar tactics back in May 1970. Now, however, the battle had become fiercer. The stakes were higher, as the captains of industrial capital sought desperately to hide the increasingly obvious shame of Minamata disease.

14. THE MINAMATA
DISEASE CENTER

As THE KUMAMOTO TRIAL drew toward a close, the patients who had chosen to attempt direct negotiations with Chisso in Tokyo saw their own heated battle near its end. So much of the patients' energy had been poured into these struggles. What would become of the patients afterward? For most of the world, the conclusion of the trial and of the battle for direct negotiations would signal the end of the entire Minamata-disease issue. The patients would be forgotten, and the people of Minamata would do their best to ensure that the patients stirred up no more unwelcome publicity or trouble.

But the end of the trial and the direct-negotiations struggle would not mean the end of the patients' personal battle against Minamata disease. This was a battle they would have to fight the rest of their lives. It is not surprising that many of the patients wanted to prolong both the trial and the negotiations.

Michiko keenly felt the patients' anxiety. There must be some way they could find peace. Why not, she thought, build a place where they could meet without shame, a place where they could receive treatment, a place that would provide them with work? Such a place would further strengthen the solidarity of the patients, already linked by their common misfortune, and would provide a base from which to combat any future attempts to contain and isolate them. Thus was born the idea of the Minamata Disease Center Soshisha (literally, "Mutual Consideration Society").

For years Michiko and Keikichi Honda had dreamed of such a center. With the help of the Association to Indict, Rokuro Hidaka, Ken'ichi Tanigawa, and other intellectuals who had spoken out in behalf of the patients, a committee was set up to oversee its construction. An outline of the proposal for the center, along with an appeal for financial support, was published in the June 1972 issue of *Kokuhatsu* in conjunction with the dispatch of two patients, Tsuginori Hamamoto and Shinobu Sakamoto, to the United Nations Conference on the Human Environment, held in Stockholm that month. On the evening of September 6, after one of the final trial sessions in Kumamoto City, Honda discussed the proposal in more detail with some of the patients. They listened with both hope and misgivings, unsure whether to allow themselves to believe in the possibility of such a thing after all that they had suffered.

The center must not remain merely a dream, Michiko resolved. To reinforce her determination, she tacked up a large blueprint of the proposed center on a wall at home. Fortunately, contributions began flowing in. The money enabled the purchase of a plot of land on a hillside overlooking the Shiranui Sea, the island of Koijishima, and the Amakusa Islands.

Wrote Hidaka in the October issue of *Kokuhatsu:*

It is very difficult for those once driven from their homeland ever to return. Yet return they must, for unless they do, all that they have suffered will have been meaningless. There is also a danger that the patients will gradually lose touch with one another, drifting apart as they concentrate on making ends meet with the help of compensation. The Minamata Disease Center Soshisha should help prevent that.

He had first heard about the idea of the center from Michiko in the spring of 1972. That fall, they met with a number of others to discuss plans. Michiko's zeal was infectious, enabling Hidaka to visualize the center almost as clearly as she did. He painted a vivid picture of all that Michiko wished the center to stand for:

> Pollution cases tend to revolve around the issue of compensation. Such cases will probably be resolved quite quickly in the future. After all, once the money's paid everything can be forgotten. But the whole point of the Minamata movement should be to fight this kind of complacent reasoning. Money alone doesn't solve the issue and mustn't be allowed to. The center should become a symbol of this philosophy.
>
> Another function of the center should be to provide a home for the patients, a place where they can find peace of mind and body. The point isn't to spend a lot of money building the center but rather to ensure that it will meet this important need. It should be a comfortable place, a homey place, not a fancy building made of synthetic materials.

When completed, the center was to be managed by the young people who had kept vigil in the tent pitched outside Chisso's Tokyo headquarters. These youths were not mere leftist ideologues. They had a deep respect for the sanctity of life and were appalled by Chisso's irresponsible destruction of human life. They had looked into the abyss of despair that Michiko had so eloquently portrayed in her writings and had been motivated to join the patients' battle, one that transcended all differences of philosophy and ideology.

These dedicated young people included students who had left their universities, disillusioned with the lifeless mass-produced education they were being offered; corporate employees who had left their jobs, reluctant to sell their souls any longer to the company; young women who had run away from comfortable, complacent families. They were content with simple food and rough clothing, and demanded no payment for their work. They gave of themselves unstintingly. To the patients, their selfless dedication was like the life-giving water of an oasis. These young men and women had proved especially helpful during the long and difficult attempt to initiate direct negotiations in Tokyo.

The young supporters and their life in the tent were vividly described in an article in *Kokuhatsu:*

As the days go by, it is increasingly clear that the tent in which the patients' supporters are staging their sit-in outside Chisso headquarters is an important symbol of the fight for direct negotiations and must be guarded and maintained at all costs. The volunteers awake around 7:00 A.M. and immediately start cleaning the entrance to the [Chisso] building, their tent, and the surrounding area. After this is done, they assemble for calisthenics and then jog around the Marunouchi business district.

After jogging, they scatter to their posts in front of Chisso headquarters and Industrial Bank of Japan (one of Chisso's major shareholders) to distribute leaflets. Titled the *Nikkan Chisso* [a play on words that can be translated roughly as the "Daily Shame"], these leaflets are daily updates on the confrontation with Chisso. Their content is also written up on a board to be read by passersby. A few people stay in the tent to clean it and prepare for the patients who will be coming from their dormitory elsewhere in the city. Only after all these chores are done do the volunteers take time to eat breakfast, which is served in shifts.

Morning presents a scene of busy activity in front of Chisso headquarters. On the sidewalk next to the tent, two young people sell a wide range of pamphlets and other literature on the Minamata struggle that are displayed on a straw mat. There are many visitors to the tent, people bringing donations of money and other items. The names of the donors are carefully recorded, as are the amounts of money and the nature of the other gifts. Several young people are kept busy welcoming the visitors and keeping the books. In one corner two others are busy writing leaflets.

When the sun is high and everyone has eaten lunch, the young people accompany the patients into Chisso headquarters to begin the daily confrontation with Chisso's reluctant executives. This is the moment everyone has been waiting for.

"Come out, Mr. Tsuchiya," calls one of the patients, referring to Chisso's director of general affairs. He does not appear, however. Instead Kawashima, head of Chisso's security force, walks up to the barricade of bars. The patients unleash their anger at Chisso. At first Kawashima is calm, but soon his voice rises in frustration and he begins screaming unintelligibly. He makes no sense, and the patients burst out laughing. Their supporters join in. Someone bangs on the bars with a hammer. Someone else turns on a tape recording introducing the families of the patients. The group chants anti-Chisso slogans and finally leaves. This ritual takes place daily in front of the barricade on the fourth floor of Chisso headquarters.

After seeing the patients back to their dormitory, the volunteers scatter throughout the city to collect donations. Two or three remain to guard the tent. The canvassing lasts for two hours.

There is a meeting at 8:00 P.M., after everyone has returned to the tent. Close to thirty young people crowd into the tent to discuss everything from the day's events to the supplies that need to be bought. All decisions are made together, and all actions are carried out together: this is the volunteers' guiding principle.

At last there is some free time. Some of the volunteers go to coffeehouses, others to the public bath. On good days, the volunteers gather in the tent for drinks and conversation. They are well disciplined, however, and are in bed by 11:00 P.M.

Such is a day in the life of the tent volunteers.

15. Verdict and Aftermath

For almost four years the patients who had chosen to fight in the courts had traveled from Minamata to the courthouse in Kumamoto City to attend the trial sessions. Finally the day on which the verdict was to be handed down drew near: March 20, 1973.

This day would be a major milestone in the patients' long battle for recognition of their suffering, but they also knew that no amount of monetary compensation could make up for what they had lost over the years. For many, the imminent conclusion of the trial stirred up bitter memories of loved ones who had died in pain; of the evil disease that had ravaged their own bodies; of the Shiranui Sea, once the source of their livelihood, now poisoned by mercury; of prejudice and discrimination.

Whatever the outcome of the trial, the patients knew it would not bring them peace. They still seethed with anger and frustration with Chisso. The formalized routine of the courtroom could not satisfy their need to vent their anger. The trial was at best only an indirect means of talking to Chisso, they felt. Some of them therefore resolved that as soon as the trial was over they would go to Tokyo to join the patients who were negotiating directly with the company.

To Michiko, the trial had the brittle artificiality of a second-rate drama: the absurdity of ordering a woman out of the courtroom when the child she was holding, a congenital victim of Minamata disease, uttered involuntary cries; the courtroom histrionics, such as the anachronistic custom of prohibiting note taking; the pompous posturing of the defendants and their lawyers. There was something about the trial that got on the patients' nerves. That their post-trial plans meant more to them than the outcome of the trial itself spoke eloquently of the extent of the Minamata tragedy and the limits of the law. The patients' own lawyers, however, could not comprehend this. They planned a meeting on the day of the verdict to celebrate their anticipated victory. They obviously wanted to impress upon the public that this was a triumph for the Communist Party. It was with great difficulty that Michiko persuaded them to forgo the event.

"To plaintiff Eizo Watanabe, eleven million yen . . . ; to plaintiff Tamotsu Watanabe, six million six hundred thousand yen. . . ." It was the morning of March 20, and Kumamoto District Court Judge Jiro Saito was reading the verdict. The name of each plaintiff was intoned and the amount of compensation, the price of a life, decreed.

The verdict harshly condemned Chisso's negligence. The judge declared that although, in operating one of the leading chemical plants in Japan, Chisso had a responsibility to ensure the highest safety standards, it had persisted for years in draining untreated waste water that included poisonous mercury into the Shiranui Sea, in gross negligence of the danger this presented to the health and lives of local residents. He also criticized Chisso's early attempts to hush up the problem with "condolence gifts," saying that the amount distributed was paltry even by the standards for monetary compensation of that time. He added that Chisso's attempt to take advantage of the patients' ignorance and its failure to compensate them properly constituted a blatant "violation of public order and conscience" and that therefore those payments were invalid.

At long last, almost twenty years after the first confirmed case of Minamata disease, Chisso was being held legally accountable for its negligence.

As the verdict was read, Michiko sat quietly in a corner of the courtroom. Despite their victory, the trial did not satisfy the patients' needs, and Michiko could not summon up much excitement over the verdict. She had shared the patients' suffering since 1959. No amount of money, she knew, could heal their wounded souls. Michiko and the patients had poured all their energy into this trial. They had achieved their goal of having Chisso publicly declared accountable for its deeds. But their victory seemed strangely hollow. They had challenged the Chisso giant on a legal battleground recognized by all. It had been imperative that they win; failure to do so would have plunged them into a bottomless abyss of despair. But winning only opened the way to the next battlefield, for this was a war without end.

The reading of the verdict did not alleviate the gloomy atmosphere in the courtroom. The patients stood as the judge left the room. Outside in the bright sun reporters and photographers scuttled about preparing to record the momentous occasion. The spacious plaza in front of the courthouse was filled with patients' supporters and black banners bearing the white character *on*.

The plaintiffs emerged, carrying photographs of family members lost to the disease. There was scattered applause, then silence: no cheers, no words of congratulation. In her mother's arms, Tomoko Kamimura croaked mindlessly: "Ah, ah." Her voice echoed through the plaza. "This child was priced at eighteen million yen," said her mother, sobbing. "But she'll never be normal." Unmindful of her mother's tears, Tomoko called out again: "Ah, ah." The black banners fluttered in the breeze.

Cameras clicked, and someone thrust a microphone in front of a patient's face. "Tell us your impressions. How do you feel about the victory?" The patient dabbed at her eyes with a handkerchief. She could not speak. Some of the Communist Party–affiliated lawyers appeared suddenly and posed at her side, very conscious of the television cameras. Their complacent expressions irritated Michiko. There were so many like them, she thought, always hovering around the patients who received the most media attention. They just wanted to be in the limelight; no wonder they had been so insensitive to the patients' true feelings and desires.

It was on this day that the Association to Indict announced that it was severing all ties with the lawyers, who wanted to join forces with the patients who were conducting direct negotiations with Chisso in Tokyo. The association charged that the lawyers had not really applied themselves to the patients' case and had tried to claim credit for the idea of corporate responsibility when, in fact, the concept had been worked out by others. The patients distrusted the lawyers and questioned their motives. They did not need the lawyers on their side; they and their supporters would continue the fight on their own. The document the association presented to the lawyers read in part:

> Countless times over the past four years we had to grit our teeth at things the patients' lawyers said and did.
>
> We were able to continue the struggle during the trial only because of the patients' indomitable fighting spirit, their supporters' dedication, and nationwide public opinion against pollution. We put up with the lawyers only because we feared disrupting the trial proceedings. Now, however, without consulting the patients and their families, these lawyers are planning to involve themselves with the patients' collective bargaining with Chisso and to disrupt the course of the Minamata-disease struggle. In view of the lawyers' plan to continue "guiding" the "ignorant" patients after the trial has ended, we cannot help feeling that our struggle is in grave danger of collapsing. . . .
>
> We repudiate any outside "guidance" of the patients in their own battle. For four years we consistently supported the patients' struggle in court, even though we sometimes had to fight off police pressure. From the beginning we have empathized with the patients' anger at Chisso's crude attempts to denigrate them and to deny the tragedy of Minamata disease, and we wholeheartedly support their tenacious struggle.
>
> We cannot condone attempts to exploit this struggle in order to further the interests of a particular political party. We are committed to standing by the patients in their endless battle, no matter how bitter and vicious it may be.

✧

"The money awarded at the trial only pays for what we have suffered so far. Now we need money to live on. Say you'll take care of us until we die!" Some of the patients who had sued Chisso, headed by Kawamoto's close friend Yoshiharu Tanoue, had arrived in Tokyo to join those involved in direct negotiations. The combined group, calling itself the Tokyo Chisso Negotiating Team, had presented Chisso's president with a pledge and were demanding that he sign it. The date was March 22, two days after the Kumamoto verdict. They felt a certain bitter satisfaction in this action. In 1959 Chisso had made so many patients sign the "condolence gift" agreement. Now they were applying the same kind of pressure to Chisso.

This was the first time Chisso's executives had agreed to allow the press to observe the negotiations. Michiko recalled the first negotiating session, held at the Mikasaya inn in Yunoko. At that time they had been adamant that the press be kept out. Now here they sat looking politely attentive.

The meeting began with Tanoue's reading of the pledge:

March 22, 1973

To Yoshiharu Tanoue, leader of the team negotiating with Chisso headquarters:

Chisso Corporation has declared that it will not appeal the ruling handed down by the Kumamoto District Court on March 20, 1973. In accordance with this, we accept all responsibility arising from the court's verdict and pledge that we will in good faith assume responsibility hereafter for making compensation for all matters having to do with Minamata disease.

Ken'ichi Shimada
President
Chisso Corporation

"Ah, I see you've worded it 'in good faith,'" responded Shimada politely. "Couldn't we change that to 'to the best of our ability'?" He could not sign the pledge, he added, unless the wording was changed.

Takae Sakamoto broke in: "You know, sir, I took sick when I was seventeen. I'm past thirty now, and I'll never be able to marry. But I still have to live, you know. I'm not asking much: just that you pay my monthly living costs. The money the court's making you pay, that only covers the more than ten years I've suffered since I was seventeen. I don't know how much longer I'm going to live. I just want you to promise I'll be taken care of. That's not asking too much, is it?"

Shimada replied that the company would go bankrupt if it promised to look after everyone. "And then what would happen to patients who come later? Don't you care?"

Dragging his useless leg, Tsuginori Hamamoto approached the negotiating table and pounded on it with his fist: "If you want to go that far, then so will I. Give me back my body the way it used to be. That's more to the point, don't you think? We don't need money. Just give me back my father and my mother."

Tanoue joined in: "Yes, do that and you owe us nothing more. This is all such a bother to you. Everything will be over and done with if you just do that."

Mitsuo Onoue tried to speak, but his vocal cords were so badly damaged that no one could make out what he was saying. His wife, Haru, interpreted: "He's telling you to listen carefully, Mr. President. The money you've given us is going to run out eventually. Now the court's handed down its ruling. So please sign the pledge. I ask you, too. Please sign the pledge and put your seal to it. You know, my husband used to be a master barber. He was especially good at shaving beards. He's been bedridden seventeen years, and all he can eat is rice mixed with fish —cat food. He's too embarrassed to eat in front of other people. I've fed him for the past seventeen years. Please, he's asking you to sign the pledge."

Shinobu Sakamoto cried out in tears, "Come on, put your seal on it!"

Fumiyo Hamamoto spoke up: "If you can return our bodies to what they once were, you don't have to sign. You don't have to pay the money the court says you're supposed to. We want our parents back again, alive. We want our children back again, alive. I'm not married; I've never even been in love. Because of Minamata disease. Why are we born? It can't be just to get sick and be paid money and then die."

"That's why I'm saying 'to the best of our ability,'" Shimada replied.

The patients would not give up. They alternately begged and demanded that Shimada sign the pledge.

"You know," said Fumiko Hiyoshi, "there can't be good faith unless both sides trust each other. But Chisso hasn't done anything so far to make us trust it. The patients are determined that this time, at least, they're not going to be tricked. So if you're really sincere, why don't you sign the pledge? I ask you as one human being to another. I beg you on my knees." So saying, she sank to her knees and bowed before Shimada.

The Chisso executives were embarrassed. "Now, now, Mrs. Hiyoshi. To do such a thing . . ."

Shimada tried to lift her to her feet, but she resisted. "This is how much you are mistrusted," she said. "There's only one way to win their trust. And this is it," she said, pointing to the pledge.

"That's right," the patients chorused.

At a loss, Shimada turned once again to Hiyoshi. "Please, please stand up. Well, if you won't, then I will kneel on the floor, too. Since you go that far, Mrs. Hiyoshi, I agree. I will sign the pledge."

Seeing their president kneeling on the floor, the other Chisso executives reluctantly followed suit.

Before long, however, Shimada's pledge was broken. At the negotiating session on April 11 Chisso flatly refused to pay the patients any further compensation. After all, the company argued, the patients had not appealed the Kumamoto District Court verdict, so they must have been satisfied with it. Michiko was not really surprised by Chisso's betrayal, however, since Shimada had been coerced into making the pledge in the first place.

"If you think we're satisfied with the court's ruling, we'll give you back your money," the patients declared. Seventeen patients' bankbooks, along with ¥18 million in cash (Mayumi Sakamoto's share), were handed to Shimada. "Just give us back our health," they said.

Taken aback by this unexpected move, the Chisso executives could only protest feebly. After several hours of fruitless discussion, the executives signed a receipt for the bankbooks and cash and agreed to review their stand on the matter.

Yet far from reviewing the matter, Chisso decided to disappear. On May 5—Children's Day, a national holiday—the patients gathered as usual on the fourth floor of Chisso's Tokyo headquarters. The quiet was suddenly broken as a stream of Chisso employees and workmen pushed past the patients into the Chisso offices. They reappeared carrying boxes of documents, which they loaded onto two large trucks waiting outside the building. Before the patients grasped what was happening, they were gone.

Thereafter, no Chisso employee set foot in the building. The company seemed to have evaporated. The patients waited for seventy days, but not a single Chisso employee appeared. Who would have thought that a company capitalized at ¥8 billion would choose to disappear rather than negotiate with a few victims of its own negligence?

The long vigil in the empty building was hard on the patients. A full year and a half had passed since they had come to Tokyo, yet they had achieved so little. And where were things to go from here? Michiko sensed that the patients were fast approaching the limit of their endurance. The tide was ebbing. But surely Chisso was feeling just as frustrated. With all avenues of escape cut off, the corporation must be seeking someone to mediate the dispute.

It was as Michiko had guessed: Chisso did not return to the negotiating table until it had found a mediator. On July 9 Chisso and the patients signed a compensation agreement at the Environment Agency, witnessed by Environment Agency Director General Takeo Miki and Kumamoto Prefecture Governor Issei

Sawada. The ceremony marked the end of a year and eight months of dogged struggle.

This was not the conclusion envisioned by the patients. They had tried hard to get Chisso to negotiate directly, but Michiko knew the year and eight months had taken its toll. The stalemate had dragged on too long; the patients, and Michiko herself, were physically and emotionally exhausted. Was their frustration to be tamped down once more by a mere ceremony?

Reporters crowded against them and cameras flashed incessantly. Tanoue took up a brush and, his hand shaking, signed the document. Kawamoto pressed the negotiating group's seal onto the paper. Akira Noguchi, a Chisso director, signed for Shimada, who was ill. Next the witnesses signed. The whole thing was over in twenty minutes.

Still, thought Michiko, this perfunctory occasion could be regarded as another milestone in the patients' endless struggle. Chisso had been compelled to make several costly concessions. For one thing, it could no longer insist that the first Minamata-disease patients be treated differently from those found to have the disease later. Under the present agreement, Chisso was obliged to compensate all patients, regardless of when they were certified, in line with the compensation stipulated in the Kumamoto trial. Furthermore, Chisso accepted full responsibility for the tragedy and expressed its regret. This formal apology was some consolation to Michiko and the patients, for Chisso had consistently tried to avoid acknowledging its responsibility.

The main points of the apology can be summarized as follows: Chisso acknowledges that it directly caused Minamata disease by failing to treat its factory wastes properly and by discharging poisonous substances into the Shiranui Sea. Chisso sincerely regrets its failure, following the official identification of Minamata disease, to take immediate measures to curb the damage, elucidate the cause of the disease, and offer help to the patients. Chisso acknowledges that the problem was greatly aggravated by its reluctance to act even after the cause of the disease was confirmed. Chisso sincerely apologizes for the pressure it has exerted on Minamata-disease patients and for its role in aggravating their suffering by encouraging the local community to discriminate against them. Chisso also apologizes for disturbing the public peace in its efforts to evade responsibility and to prolong the negotiating process with the patients. Because of Chisso's failure to acknowledge the existence of patients throughout the region of the Shiranui Sea and to make active efforts to seek them out, the full extent of the disease is still not known. Chisso promises to apply all its resources henceforth to seeking out and aiding victims of the disease whose existence has not yet been acknowledged.

The battle was over. The tent that had stood so long in front of Chisso's Tokyo headquarters was to be taken down. On July 12, about seventy people gathered in front of Chisso headquarters for a final farewell. The tent had been home to many of the patients' supporters for over a year and a half, but little energy was wasted on sentimental goodbyes. The young volunteers set about striking the tent with cheerful efficiency. Someone picked up a dogeared copy of *Paradise of the Bitter Sea* and tucked it carefully into a knapsack.

Altogether, about two hundred young people had stayed in this tent since it had been raised in December 1971. Now they scattered, some to universities, others to jobs, still others to Minamata; but all retained vivid memories of the long struggle.

When Michiko had been thrown out of the Chisso building that cold winter night, which seemed so long ago now, she had found refuge in the tent. This tent was a living, breathing entity, she thought. She had expected the young people who had set it up to use it for only a month or two. Who could have imagined it would remain standing so long? Only the vigor of youth could have kept it there. The tent had been an oasis in the Tokyo desert.

Standing where the tent had been, Kawamoto was clearly full of emotion as he addressed the group: "We could never have fought so long without the support of you young ones. Now the battle moves back to Minamata. Thank you all. The canvas tent is gone, but the tent of hope and courage remains in our hearts."

One by one, scenes from the long struggle flashed before Michiko's eyes. Yes, the tent will remain in our hearts, she thought, a symbol of refuge and encouragement for the times of trouble that are still before us. She bade farewell to the volunteers and left with the patients to return to Minamata.

The drawn-out process of direct negotiations seemed to many of the volunteer supporters to have been ignited by the flaming convergence of Kawamoto's smoldering hatred for Chisso and Michiko's jealous guardianship of the dead souls of the Shiranui Sea. Yet Michiko had no sense of having played a major role. She knew only that she continued to be driven by the same need to right a dreadful wrong that had overtaken her upon her first sight of a Minamata-disease patient in May 1959. She was like an incarnation of the patients' suffering souls, cursing Chisso for the thoughtless havoc it had wreaked upon the once-peaceful Shiranui Sea, calling out dire warnings against the way in which science and technology had violated the sanctity of human life.

The driving force within Michiko spoke through her many writings on Minamata disease and the Minamata-disease patients. Every bit of money she received from publishing her works went into the patients' war chest. Her writings thus provided invaluable support, both psychological and material.

She disliked awards of any kind, but she was finally prevailed upon to accept the Ramon Magsaysay Prize, awarded to her in August 1973 for her literary achievements. Having turned down the Oya Prize and a literary award from the *Kumamoto Nichinichi Shimbun*, she did not see why she should accept the Magsaysay Prize, either, but friends urged her to do so. The $10,000 in prize money, she was reminded, could be used to help build the Minamata Disease Center Soshisha. Thinking it over, she realized that circumstances had changed considerably since her refusal of the Oya Prize in 1970. The trial was over, and the direct negotiations had finally been concluded; there was now a momentary lull in the battle.

There was another reason she decided to accept the Magsaysay Prize. The presentation ceremony would be held in Manila, and on the way home she could stop off in Malaysia to meet some of the *karayuki-san* who had left the Amakusa Islands for Southeast Asia so long ago. The *karayuki-san* were Japanese women who had been shipped off to other Asian countries before World War II to work as prostitutes. A large number had gone from Amakusa, sold into prostitution by families too poor to keep them. Many of these same families had been among the first affected by Minamata disease. Michiko did indeed meet a former *karayuki-san,* now an old woman living in Malaysia, and heard her sad story. The prize money left after deducting the expenses for this detour went directly into the fund for the center. Finally, in April 1974, Michiko saw her dream realized. The center was built just as she had envisioned, overlooking the Shiranui Sea and the Amakusa Islands.

Meanwhile, Michiko returned to writing full time, renting a small office in Kumamoto City. She spent weekdays there and weekends in Minamata with her husband and mother. The office provided a much-needed refuge from the distractions of Minamata. Here she could concentrate on the interrupted first sequel to *Paradise of the Bitter Sea,* a biography of Itsue Takamure, and other writing projects. This new life was far from idyllic, however, for Michiko found her work interrupted frequently by patients' problems.

16. LAW VERSUS JUSTICE

THE END OF THE TRIAL and the direct negotiations by no means quenched the smoldering embers of the Minamata flame. On January 13, 1975, Teruo Kawamoto was found guilty of five counts of infliction of bodily injury on Chisso employees, fined ¥50,000, and given a one-year suspended sentence. His lawyers promptly appealed, claiming that the verdict contravened "the government's policy of providing relief for the victims of industrial pollution."

Upon hearing the verdict, thirty patients and family members and more than a hundred young supporters who had gathered in front of the Tokyo District Court began chanting, "Down with the reactionary verdict!" They persisted despite orders to cease. The same day, Kawamoto and his sympathizers held a protest rally. Gazing up at the forest of black *on* banners, Kawamoto addressed the crowd: "The complicity of the national and prefectural governments was a major factor in the tragedy of Minamata disease. Now we know the courts, too, are on the side of the corporations." He then announced his decision to appeal.

The patients' resentment boiled over. "It's unforgivable that we should be charged with crimes while the real criminal gets off scot-free." By this time 150 people had died from Chisso's poisonous mercury. It was resolved at the rally to counterattack by charging Kiichi Nishioka, Chisso president from 1958 to 1964, and Eiichi Nishida, manager of the Minamata plant from 1957 to 1960, with homicide and infliction of bodily injury. Charges were filed that very day.

Until this time, the patients had refrained from retaliating against Chisso's charges to avoid diverting attention from the central issue, the tragedy of Minamata disease itself. But they could not let Chisso get away with having a victim of mercury poisoning branded a criminal. Michiko sighed. Another hard struggle begins, she thought.

"Now that Chisso executives have been charged with homicide, the police have begun investigating the company. What do you think of that?" a reporter asked Michiko. She only replied, "I'm too dispirited even to talk about it." When Michiko thought about how the police had helped Chisso apply pressure to the patients, she could not see how anything could come of an investigation of Chisso now. Every encounter with the police so far had left a bitter aftertaste: when the police had stepped in to quash the fishers' protests; when they had applied subtle tactics of discouragement to get people to rescind their applications for certification as patients; when they had arrested supporters for disrupting the proceedings of the Compensation Committee; when they had conducted their heavy-handed investigation of Kawamoto.

The police had consistently ignored the mass poisoning taking place before their very eyes, instead exerting relentless pressure on the victims. It was clear, thought Michiko, whom they were maintaining so-called law and order for. The police had never helped the patients; why should the patients trust the police now? As far as the Minamata issue was concerned, the police certainly seemed more intent on suppressing the weak to protect the strong than the reverse.

The patients' frustration and anger with the police and their tactics finally exploded on July 10, 1975, at a meeting between representatives of the patients and officers of the Kumamoto prefectural police. The meeting took place at the Minamata Disease Center Soshisha, in a room enshrining the spirits of the 150 people who had already died of Minamata disease. Four police officers, headed by Crime Prevention Division Director Takeo

Sakurai, had come to ask the patients to cooperate with the police investigation of the patients in connection with the patients' charges against Chisso executives. Representing the patients were thirty or so members of the League of Minamata Disease Patients (the successor to the Tokyo Chisso Negotiating Team), including the group's representative, Tsuginori Hamamoto.

Hamamoto opened the meeting with a statement rebuking the prefectural police: "If the prefectural police headquarters had taken proper action against Chisso a long time ago, the damage and loss caused by Minamata disease could have been minimized. Now that we've charged Chisso executives with homicide and infliction of bodily injury, the police are investigating us first, when Chisso should be their target. This just gives Chisso time to destroy crucial evidence. We cannot condone such an approach."

"Whom we decide to investigate first is our business; it's not your place to tell us how to do our job. We intend to clarify the facts of the case on the basis of information collected from both sides," responded Sakurai.

"A lot of people have suffered and died on account of the poisonous wastes from the Chisso plant. Everyone's known this for a long time now. The Kumamoto trial concluded that Chisso was at fault, yet the police have done nothing up to now."

"That's not true. We've been investigating Minamata disease for a quite a while. We have stacks of documents on the case. We've investigated every single suspicious point, just as we would in a robbery."

"I don't know what you've been investigating, but it certainly hasn't been Chisso. One of the executives at Chisso told us so himself. He said you hadn't come once to investigate them."

"Did he really say that?"

"He sure did. He's one of their directors; I can even tell you his name."

Sakurai made no reply.

"Why do you lie to us, when you haven't investigated Chisso even once?"

Silence.

"You've been on our backs all the time. Every time patients went to a trial session, there you were. You've been focusing only on us."

"Now, now. We will certainly base the present investigation on objective evaluation of the data. We'll be coming around to your homes to ask some questions, and we ask for your cooperation. The Japanese police are the best in the world, you know. Please trust us."

Someone called out, "Yeah, the Japanese police are the best in the world when it comes to putting down the weak." The room broke into laughter, quickly replaced by a glum silence.

Soon after that, something happened that seemed to confirm the patients' feeling that the police were bent on harassing them. Two patients awaiting certification and two supporters were arrested without warning.

According to *Minamata* (formerly *Kokuhatsu;* the publication was renamed in September 1973), it all began on September 25, 1975, when 150 members of the Council of Applicants for Certification as Minamata Disease Patients (formed in August 1974) and the League of Minamata Disease Patients traveled by bus from Minamata to Kumamoto City to visit the Kumamoto Prefecture Special Committee on Pollution Countermeasures. Earlier, on August 7, the committee's chairman, Kunio Sugimura, had complained to the Environment Agency that many spurious patients were applying for certification in the hope of getting their hands on compensation money and that the Certification Board was having a hard time weeding out the false patients. The 150 patients, family members, and supporters went to Kumamoto City to protest Sugimura's remarks.

When the protesters arrived at the prefectural assembly hall, they found more than thirty plainclothes police awaiting them. Undaunted, the protesters divided into two groups. One went to the prefectural police headquarters to file a charge of slander against Sugimura, while the other entered the prefectural assembly building to demand that Sugimura apologize for his remarks before the committee. In response, Sugimura read a prepared statement to the committee in a voice so low the protesters could hardly hear it: "I regret that a misunderstanding has arisen from mistaken reports of my remarks." He then announced the committee meeting adjourned and stood up to leave the room.

"Are you trying to make fools of us? Come on, take responsibility for your own words!" Shouts of protest followed Sugimura, now protected by a contingent of plainclothes police, as he walked to another room about thirty meters away. The police prevented the patients from following. Stymied, the protesters gave up and returned to Minamata, vowing that they would not let Sugimura get away with this.

Who would have thought this incident would lead to four of them being arrested on suspicion of inflicting bodily injury and obstructing the performance of official duties?

Wind and rain lashed Minamata on the morning of October 7. More than twenty police vehicles, carrying 140 policemen, sped through the downpour. They scattered to the homes of Minamata-disease patients Noboru Sakamoto and Masato Ogata, the office of the Council of Applicants, the Minamata Disease Center Soshisha, and the home of supporter Yuko Nakamura. It was just after 6:00 A.M.

The Sakamotos' two elementary school children were just waking up. Startled by a commotion outside, the family opened the door to see policemen lined up at one-meter intervals around the house. As Noboru Sakamoto rubbed his eyes in amazement, several policemen pushed their way into the house and announced, "You are under arrest for the September 25 incident." Handcuffs were clamped on his wrists. What, thought Sakamoto in confusion, happened on September 25? With no further explanation he was pulled out of the house, pushed into a police car, and whisked away in the rain. Ignoring Sakamoto's wife, the police searched the house, ostensibly in search of evidence. When they finally left, they took with them copies of *Kokuhatsu, Minamata,* and *Paradise of the Bitter Sea.*

The police searched six locations in this manner, arresting Sakamoto, Ogata, Nakamura, and, in Kumamoto City, supporter Hiroshi Moriyama. The arrests naturally caused an uproar. Rokuro Hidaka, Ineko Sata, Junji Kinoshita, and Michio Matsuda were among the fifty-five intellectuals who immediately issued a public protest against the arrests.

"We were framed," said Sakamoto when he later described what had happened:

> There's no doubt about it, we were framed. The police knew exactly how many patients boarded the buses [to Kumamoto City]. When Sugimura left the [committee] room that day, I tried to follow him, but one of the plainclothes police stuck out his foot and tripped me. When I complained, he hid his face behind his walkie-talkie and ran off.
>
> The public prosecutors tried to scare me. "You're going to lose this one anyway," they told me. "A man of your age, and with a family, too. Why are you hanging around with these student radicals?" It's obvious they were out to smash the Council of Applicants.
>
> On October 13 I went into convulsions and threw up everything I'd eaten. Until October 16 I lived on tea and water. The police would only bring a surgeon to see me. When they finally took me to the Red Cross hospital, the doctors there just shook their heads and said they didn't know anything about Minamata disease. It was pretty rough treatment.

On October 17 Sakamoto and the three others were indicted on the charge of inflicting bodily injury during the September 25 protest. Clearly they had been unjustly accused, thought Michiko angrily. This had to be made clear at their trial. She phoned Hidaka in Tokyo. Could he, she asked, organize an investigation to dig out the facts of the case? Hidaka agreed. On October 24 he arrived in Kumamoto City leading a team that included Tokyo University Professor Michio Inaba, Tokyo University of Economics Associate Professor Norio Tamura, and Michiko Nakajima, a lawyer. The team reported its findings in the January 1976 issue of *Minamata*. There was a strong likelihood that the accusations against the patients were false, part of a politically motivated plot to discredit the patients, said the report:

The arrests made the patients and their supporters appear to be brutal criminals, when what had actually happened was too minor to warrant prosecution. . . . Only a deliberate attempt to exert psychological and social pressure on the Council of Applicants can explain the action. . . . It would also explain why so much time and energy has been spent questioning those arrested about the council. Already more than three thousand people have applied for certification. For Chisso and the government, this is a grave issue, for it is in their interest to keep the number of certifications to a minimum and to erase the issue of Minamata disease from public awareness as soon as possible. . . .

The investigating team cannot help suspecting that the prefectural police are colluding [with Chisso and the government] instead of trying, as fellow human beings, to understand the suffering of the patients and their families. The authorities are doing nothing to alleviate this suffering. . . . If those representing Chisso and the government had any conscience at all, they would surely realize that paying compensation is the very least they could do.

The Kumamoto prefectural authorities have announced that at the present rate, it will take another twenty-three years to process the more than three thousand applications for certification. In the meantime, the old will die, and the other patients will surely lose all hope. Who created this situation? . . .

When we consider this basic question, we are forced to conclude that the present arrests and indictments represent a great social injustice.

Meanwhile, the government decided to prop up Chisso with an infusion of about ¥2 billion. And somewhere along the line the patients' criminal charges against Chisso executives had been reduced from "homicide and infliction of bodily injury" to "infliction of death and bodily injury caused by negligence in the conduct of business." The police claimed they could find no evidence of criminal intent on Chisso's part, and the defendants,

Yoshioka and Nishida, denied having been aware of the health hazard caused by the discharge of effluent into the sea.

Yet the written apology Chisso executives had made to the patients who were demanding direct negotiations had clearly stated that Chisso acknowledged having directly caused Minamata disease by failing to treat factory wastes properly and by discharging poisonous substances into the Shiranui Sea. Did the subsequent denial mean that Chisso had not meant what it had said before?

Michiko could think of at least three times that the police had had ample cause to initiate an investigation of Chisso's criminal liability for Minamata disease. The first was in 1963, when Kumamoto University researchers had discovered organic mercury in effluent from Chisso's Minamata plant. The second was in September 1968, when the Ministry of Health and Welfare had officially declared that Minamata disease was a pollution-related disease caused by Chisso effluent. The third was in March 1973, when Chisso was found guilty of gross negligence in the Kumamoto trial. It was clear who was the victim and who the perpetrator of the crime.

More than a decade had passed since Kumamoto University had pinpointed the culprit. The Ministry of Health and Welfare declaration and the Kumamoto verdict had further focused the spotlight on Chisso. Yet the police still could not bring themselves to investigate Chisso's criminal responsibility. Even when the issue was raised in the Diet, the police excused their lack of activity by muttering about insufficient evidence and the statute of limitations. What a contrast to their relentless pursuit of the patients and their supporters!

Only when the exasperated patients formally charged Chisso executives with homicide and infliction of bodily injury were the police forced to act. Even then, though, they moved with the greatest reluctance, treating a sordid crime of mass poisoning as if it were nothing more than a traffic accident.

How could anyone claim there was no criminal intent behind Chisso's actions? What about the order to halt cat experiments, revealed by Hosokawa on his deathbed? Chisso had known that cat 400 had been poisoned by effluent, yet had done nothing to stop the discharge of lethal wastes. Instead, the company had forced the patients to accept nominal "condolence gifts." What about the company's useless "purification equipment"? What about the acknowledged fact that Chisso had continued to drain untreated wastes into the sea for almost ten years after the presence of organic mercury had been confirmed? Chisso had willfully ignored Hosokawa's dire warnings. If that was not criminal intent, what was?

The police certainly were not likely to find much evidence after all these years, especially since they were not trying very hard. Chisso had had more than enough time to destroy incriminating evidence. Michiko's heart was heavy.

On May 4, 1976, Yoshioka and Nishida were indicted on charges of infliction of death and bodily injury caused by negligence in the conduct of business, and the first session of the trial was held in the Kumamoto District Court on September 22.

Michiko was pessimistic. The point of filing charges had been to show that Chisso had known about the danger of mercury poisoning and yet had chosen to do nothing. Without the charge of criminal intent, the outcome of the trial was already evident. "It's a farce. It's obvious how it's going to turn out. There's no hope for a world where you can't even tell black and white apart," lamented her friend Satoru Akazaki.

When would the patients escape from the abyss? They had done no wrong, yet two of them, along with two supporters, were threatened with imprisonment. They had to be spared this final humiliation. But that meant another long trial that they would have to win. They would need money. Once again, Michiko took pen in hand to solicit funds:

> Yesterday the world appeared bright red. Today black butterflies flutter their useless wings before my eyes. Within the red blur, through the black butterfly wings, I see glimpses of all your faces. Your faces rise and sink, rise and sink. They sink because once again I am asking for donations. How many times have I asked for your help?

I realize that raising money is a dirty business, since money is tainted with all the world's dark currents of emotion.

I am the puppeteer. From my hands dangle a doctor puppet, a policeman puppet, and a diseased puppet. A gleaming shackle is clamped to the diseased puppet's leg. "Come on now, stand up, you fake patient. You want money, eh? Well, money is metal. Here's some metal for you," says the policeman puppet, waving a pair of handcuffs. The diseased puppet shakes its head, click, click, click. The red darkness spreads.

"Put them around its neck. Around its neck," whispers the doctor puppet. The handcuffs dance around the diseased puppet's head as it swings this way and that.

Like autumn leaves, a brilliant shower of money rains down upon us. The diseased puppet and I, the puppeteer, are ashamed to be alive. Was it a bad dream or a good dream? Suddenly we start awake and realize we're in for another trial. This time the Minamata patients are being accused of being a danger to this world. This is going to require a lot of money. We're going to have to bother everyone again.

We bow deeply as the handcuffs clatter and glitter behind us. In a world with as many sorrows as there are stars, it is painful to have to beg once again for your help.

These bleak events were followed by one piece of news that seemed to promise a glimmer of light ahead. Kawamoto's second trial ended in victory. The judge even quoted Michiko's writings. The verdict was read out in the Tokyo High Court on June 14, 1977, eight years to the day after the patients who had opted for litigation had filed suit against Chisso. Kawamoto could hardly believe his ears.

"We have no words with which to describe the tragedy of Minamata disease. The police must not fall so low as to torment the weak. The indictment itself is illegal." Judge Masaji Terao not only overturned the district court's verdict of guilty but went on to rebuke Chisso for its efforts to evade responsibility for the worst case of mercury pollution in history and the authorities and public prosecutors for failing to come to the victims' aid, charging that their frivolous indictment was discriminatory and an abuse of their power. Never before had a judge passed such harsh judgment upon the prosecution. A hush fell on the court-room after he finished reading the verdict. The prosecutors were stunned.

It took Terao forty-five minutes to read the verdict. In an un-usual move, he referred directly to Michiko's writings about the Shiranui Sea: "I have also read Michiko Ishimure's most recent work, *Tsubaki no Umi no Ki* [Chronicle of the Sea of Camellias], in which she describes the beauty of the sea of Minamata be-fore it was polluted. The nation prospers, but our mountains and streams perish."

This precedent-setting verdict was front-page news. The *Asahi Shimbun* story, headlined with Terao's words "The nation prospers, but our mountains and streams perish," included a de-scription of Kawamoto and Michiko listening to the verdict be-ing read. Michiko was quoted as saying, when asked her opinion of the verdict, "It was a humane verdict, I think. But there are more than ten thousand patients. . . ."

Though Kawamoto urged the public prosecutors not to ap-peal the high court's verdict, since doing so would make the government a willing accomplice in the attempt to discredit the patients, they filed an appeal the very next day, on the grounds that the verdict challenged the very basis of prosecutorial au-thority and was unconstitutional, having overstepped the bounds of judicial authority. The case would now have to go to the Su-preme Court. The conservative Supreme Court was not likely to come down so firmly on the patients' side, but Kawamoto was determined to do his best to gain another "humane ver-dict." He immediately launched a campaign to collect one mil-lion signatures.

✧

Colorful new houses against a backdrop of tangerine groves dot the peaceful coast of the Shiranui Sea. The dilapidated homes of the fishers have disappeared, and the scene resembles that of a resort. The first thing the patients did when they received their compensation payments from Chisso was to build new homes. They were tired of cowering in hovels, hiding from society's merciless gaze. They wanted to live in ordinary houses to prove that they too were human. They were also driven by the natural desire to exorcise the aura of disease that had permeated their old homes. But their attempt to live ordinary lives like ordinary people continues to draw down on them envy and suspicion. In any case, new houses do not alleviate the patients' pain.

And how many more still live in squalid quarters? How many more along the Shiranui Sea await certification? How many are afflicted but too frightened to step forward? The mercury-poisoned waves of the Shiranui Sea continue to corrode people's hearts and bodies.

As of September 1977, more than two hundred people had died of Minamata disease, around one thousand had been certified as patients, and another four thousand were awaiting certification. But these figures represented only the tip of the iceberg. There were believed to be over ten thousand cases, and at least a hundred thousand people exposed to mercury pollution.

Minamata Bay had once been a treasure-trove of fish. Now its bed was coated in several meters of mercury-contaminated sludge. The sea will probably never revert to its former pristine condition. In fact, the national government, the prefectural government, and Chisso have already spent ¥20 billion to dredge the bay and fill it in. The voices of happy children that once echoed along its shores have long since fallen silent. An evil spirit now resides in what was once a kind and gentle sea. A national policy of prosperity at any cost has allowed a single corporation to damage the environment irreversibly. The beautiful Shiranui Sea has been sacrificed to the pursuit of profit.

AFTERWORD

"TAKAYAMA is going through the same thing Minamata went through, isn't it?" said Michiko Ishimure when I first met her, in 1974. Her words planted the seed that would eventually grow into this book. The coastal city of Minamata and the mountain city of Takayama share a bond of pain. Both have had their water poisoned, and both have had to fight callous and irresponsible authorities.

I grew up in Takayama, a lovely city nestled in the mountains of Gifu Prefecture, central Honshu, and long famous for the purity of its water. But since 1972 Takayama's citizens have been drinking water poisoned with copper. The city's rising popularity as a tourist attraction in the late 1960s strained the limits of the drinking-water supply, and city officials decided to draw additional water from the Kohachiga River, which flows from the northern Japan Alps, not realizing that there was an abandoned copper mine near the river's source. The Hiragane copper mine, at the foot of the Norikuradake mountains, just twenty-five kilometers upstream from Takayama, had been one of Japan's major copper mines in the late nineteenth and early twentieth centuries. Even now the water of the Kohachiga River is the color of verdigris near its source, and no fish or any other living creatures are to be found in its waters.

Between 1959 and 1965 there was an outbreak of a strange illness among infants living along the river. They would run a high fever, after which their heads would swell, and eventually many would die. Those who survived were brain damaged, and many had to be committed to institutions. Alarmed, a group of Takayama citizens suggested that copper poisoning was the cause and demanded that the city's drinking water be tested. Just as they had suspected, the water was found to have an inordinately high heavy-metal content. An appeal was immediately made to the local authorities to change the city's source of water.

But the city had spent over ¥1 billion on the new waterworks, and construction was almost complete. Declaring that there was no turning back now, the city opened the taps to water from the Kohachiga River on December 30, 1971. There were rumors at the time that shady dealings behind the scenes had forced this suicidal move. Once before, the Kohachiga River had been contemplated as a source of drinking water. At that time, however, tests had shown the water to contain arsenic and the plan had been abandoned. This time, however, the city officials had been so eager to maintain Takayama's tourist industry that they had chosen the same tainted river without running proper tests.

An investigative team from Nagoya University's School of Medicine had identified the infants' malady as hydrocephalus and had warned the city government that there was a direct relationship between the city's water supply and the disorder. Instead of heeding this warning, however, the city had chosen to accept the argument to the contrary of a scholar who had never even seen the river, Professor Tamon Ishibashi of Tokyo University's Faculty of Engineering. Gifu Prefecture's Sanitation Department had complied with the Takayama city officials' wishes by fabricating water-quality test results, and the Ministry of Health and Welfare had compounded the deception by accepting the figures without question and giving the go-ahead for the new waterworks.

The Kohachiga River flows into the Jinzu River. The pathologist Noboru Hagino, who in the mid-1950s identified the syndrome that came to be known as *itai itai* (ouch ouch) disease, a pollution disease caused by cadmium discharged from the Kamioka mine, situated on the upper reaches of the Jinzu, confirmed through animal experiments that copper from the Hiragane mine was a contributing factor. "It bodes ill for Takayama if the people there continue to drink this water," Hagino warned.

I was working in the Nagoya bureau of the *Asahi Shimbun* at the time of the Takayama water controversy and decided to cover the problem. Over a two-year period I gathered enough data to write a book about it, *Hametsu no Mizu* (Water of Ruin). But by the time the book was published, in November 1973, I had been transferred to Kyushu and had to observe subsequent events in Takayama from a distance. Though the book stirred interest in the issue among people in Takayama, the city authorities succeeded in muzzling all public protest except for a small citizens' movement.

While I was on Kyushu, Jun Ui, one of the first people to become involved in the Minamata issue, read my book and visited Takayama. With the help of Kiyo'o Omori, a poet and an activist in the local citizens' movement, Ui tested the water near the Hiragane mine himself. He was shocked to learn the city was providing its citizens with drinking water from a source so tainted that not a fish was to be found in its waters. "You must put a stop to the use of water from such a contaminated source before you end up with a tragedy like that of Minamata disease," he warned. Ui believed that the people of Takayama, unlike those of Minamata, still had a chance to avert disaster if they moved quickly.

After leaving Takayama, Ui lectured on the need for people to take a greater interest in the sources of their drinking water and the danger of allowing local governments to build waterworks without conducting thorough water-quality tests first. He also criticized Ishibashi for giving the Takayama authorities the go-ahead for their plan without having checked the water source himself. An authority on water-supply systems, Ishibashi emphasized the need to carry out environmental tests before deciding on a water source; yet he had approved Takayama's waterworks plan on the basis of the doctored test data the city had supplied. He had even gone so far as to say that the people of Takayama could take pride in the fine quality of their water. The city, of course, had been delighted by his support and had published his assurances in the city government's bulletin, which was distributed to everyone in Takayama.

On July 21, 1976, Omori and Ichiro Urada, the leader of the Takayama citizens' group, took part in a seminar on pollution being conducted by Ui and others at Tokyo University. There they met Teruo Kawamoto and some of the other Minamata-disease patients for the first time. They saw for themselves what polluted water had done to these people, and their concern for their own city was heightened.

The Minamata-disease patients had had to fight long and hard, and even though they had won their suit against Chisso, they continued to suffer. Omori and the others from Takayama could see that their own battle to prevent pollution was not going to be easy.

Omori told the seminar audience:

Takayama's new water purification plant resembles nothing so much as a depository for factory effluent. The heavy metals flowing in from the abandoned Hiragane mine accumulate in a settling reservoir. The sludge in this reservoir was found to contain 133 ppm of copper, 33.8 ppm of arsenic, 0.6 ppm of mercury, 30.2 ppm of lead, and 0.56 ppm of cadmium, but the Gifu Prefecture Sanitation Department suppressed these data. Every month some thirty tons of this sludge is buried within the purification plant's grounds as waste. The water we drink every day is skimmed off this sludge. The people living upstream along the Kohachiga River won't drink its water, yet this same water is piped into the homes of Takayama's citizens. A growing number of people worried about the water's polluting effects are digging wells to try to protect themselves.

The city officials and politicians refuse to acknowledge that they've made a basic error of judgment, and they have a hired scholar to abet their attempt to deceive the people. The people of Takayama are victims of an irresponsible human experiment. Our own surveys reveal that the death rate is rising among infants and the elderly in districts supplied from the new water source. Must we wait until the harm is too great to ignore? The suffering of the Minamata-disease patients may become a reality for us too if nothing is done.

The tourists crowding the quaint streets of Takayama do not seem to hear Omori's warning. Even the quiet district where I grew up is now crammed with gift shops and looks more like a movie set than part of a living, breathing town.

The people continue to drink the poisoned water, too happy about the prosperity tourism has brought them to think about what may be happening to their bodies. Takayama is doubly polluted by tourism and a suspect water supply. Meanwhile, those who know the real dangers wonder what the symptoms of "Takayama disease" will be. In Minamata, the authorities ignored the problem of Chisso's effluent for almost a decade, thereby allowing incalculable harm to be done to human beings and the environment. Will the Takayama authorities do the same? How long do they think they can keep their heads buried in the sand?

It was Michiko Ishimure who made me aware of the bond between Takayama and Minamata. I knew she had played a major part in the Minamata-disease struggle, and I wanted to interview her about Takayama's water pollution. Perhaps she would offer some encouragement to those fighting the problem. Before we met, I reread *Paradise of the Bitter Sea* and was moved once again by its vivid descriptions of the Minamata-disease patients' suffering.

I finally met Michiko early in the summer of 1974. I visited her at her office on a quiet side street in Kumamoto City. Light filtered through the leaves of the tree in the yard onto the tatami mats of a room as neat as a pin. She had obviously been reading the copy of *Water of Ruin* that I had sent her a month earlier. The book lay open on a table, under a special magnifying glass. The long years of struggle had taken their toll on her eyes. She was almost blind in the left eye and had only minimal vision in the right eye.

"If you don't get clean water in Takayama soon, the whole country may go the same way, and that will be the end of us all," she said. "I've always admired Takayama, not least because it's one of the last truly beautiful places in Japan. It's ironic that people living in such a lovely setting should be in danger from their own water supply. The authorities seem to be as determined to strangle the local citizens' movement in Takayama as in Minamata. If I didn't live so far away, I'd go to Takayama immediately to encourage the people there in their fight. But my eyes are too weak, and I have work to do here. The best I can do is support Takayama indirectly through my writings on Minamata disease."

Michiko understood the gravity of the threat to Takayama. In 1971, just before direct negotiations were to begin with Chisso, she had traveled to the Ashio copper mine, in Tochigi Prefecture, central Honshu, one of the first places in Japan to draw attention because of water pollution. She visited the site where the village of Yanaka, most heavily affected by the pollution and eventually razed by government order, had once stood and traced the movements of the great Japanese environmentalist Shozo Tanaka (1841–1913), who had championed the local residents' cause.

I was deeply moved by her declaration that she hoped she could help the people of Takayama through her writings on Minamata disease. Did I too not have a duty to take pen in hand to convey the tragedy of Minamata to the people of Takayama? Here I was, already on Kyushu. I could begin my research right away. There seemed to be a fine thread pulling me ever closer to Minamata.

One of the places I visited in the course of my research was Meisui-en, a facility for severely disabled Minamata-disease patients. There, for the first time, I saw patients born with the disease; and what I saw depressed me profoundly. These patients were by then fifteen or sixteen years old. Their arms and legs were like stiff sticks. I had arrived at lunch time and watched as the boys and girls were laid out on the tatami floor and a bib was tied around each one's neck. As the nurses spoon-fed them, the patients uttered pathetic cries: "Ah, ah." When the meal was over, I was asked to wait outside in the hall. A curtain was closed, and I learned later that one of the patients was having her diaper changed. This young woman, her breasts already filled out, cringed in shame every time she had to have someone else take care of her menstrual needs, I was told.

Before me the blue Shiranui Sea glittered in the sunlight. Because of this sea these children had been transformed into living corpses. Every aspect of Minamata disease returned to this sea, a sea that had once been mother to all who partook of her bounty but was now a bitter sea of suffering. I could feel myself drowning in waves of despair. Too great a price had been paid for industrial prosperity.

As I continued my research, talking again with Michiko and with the patients and others closely involved in the history of Minamata disease and poring over mountains of documents and papers, I realized how complex, how cruel, and how violent had been the patients' long battle. What the patients and their supporters had endured defied imagination. I was especially moved by the stories of those people, not patients themselves, who had given their all to try to pull the patients out of their abyss of misery. My greatest respect was for Michiko, who through her writings had conveyed the soul-wrenching appeals of the victims of Minamata disease with an unmatched eloquence.

The story of Minamata disease has now been told around the world, and it has come to symbolize the tragedy of wanton environmental destruction. But no one has yet attempted to convey the full story of the people behind the patients, who willingly sacrificed their own lives to support the patients' cause. To borrow an analogy of Michiko's, these were the *kurogo*, the stagehands dressed in identity-concealing black who assist actors onstage. Yet it is only because of these people that one of the most moving dramas in the dark history of our pollution of this planet continues to be told.

After a year and a half of research, I returned to Nagoya to write my account of the Minamata-disease patients' battle against the powers that be. When I first asked Michiko for permission to center the book on her, she refused, asking me to choose someone else. She preferred, as ever, to avoid the spotlight and remain on the sidelines. But in tracing the history of Minamata disease, it became obvious to me that Michiko was there every step of the way, encouraging others. To give just one example, it was her writings that opened Masazumi Harada's eyes to the plight of the victims of Minamata disease; before he read her moving descriptions, he had seen only the disease, not the suffering patients. Awakened to what was really important in medicine, Harada joined the patients in their court battle against Chisso, testifying to the unforgivable harm Chisso had inflicted upon innocent people.

Sadao Togashi of Kumamoto University, who was also involved in the Kumamoto trial and who formulated the concept of Chisso's corporate responsibility for the disaster, told me in an interview, "Minamata disease is so compelling it never lets go of your soul. I think Michiko Ishimure is the living embodiment of this quality." I agree; in no other person battling pollution have I seen such burning dedication.

Togashi also made me aware of how much the patients had suffered at the hands of their own lawyers. "The truth about that story needs to be told," he said. It was indeed an amazing story. As the lawyers revealed their communist leanings, the patients found them harder and harder to work with. Yet the patients and their supporters persevered, organizing the Minamata Disease Study Group and winning the case essentially on their own. Michiko was at the center of that battle, too. She was also there throughout the year and eight months of confrontation between the patients and Chisso in Tokyo.

As a journalist, I was ashamed to realize I had lived through the worst case of mercury poisoning in history without having comprehended the gravity and cruelty of the wounds it had inflicted on innocent lives. But this realization enabled me to persuade Michiko to allow me to build my story around her. The behind-the-scenes story—the saga of the battle against corrupt authority in a nation second to none in pollution—needed to be told to as many people as possible. My book would be one more weapon in the war we must wage to ensure that never again is there another Minamata.

I am not confident that an outsider like me can adequately convey the extreme depth of the abyss. I am grateful to Michiko, to the others who figure in this book, and to the many people whose names I have not recorded, for their cooperation. Finally, I pray that this book may be of some solace to the souls of the Minamata patients who have died, and I pray too that Takayama's "water of ruin" may become "water of rejuvenation."

CHRONOLOGY OF
MAJOR EVENTS

1906	Shitagau Noguchi establishes Sogi Electric Co.
1908	Sogi Electric's name is changed to Japan Nitrogen Fertilizer Co. (Nippon Chisso Hiryo Kabushiki Kaisha), popularly known as Chisso
July 1932	Chisso's Minamata plant begins production of acetaldehyde using mercury as a catalyst and discharging untreated wastes into Hyakken Harbor
Dec. 1946	Initial outbreak of the syndrome later named Minamata disease (acknowledged in April 1971)
Jan. 1950	Japan Nitrogen Fertilizer Co. is reorganized as New Japan Nitrogen Co.
Dec. 1953	The first person to be certified as a Minamata-disease patient exhibits symptoms (the patient died in March 1956 and was certified posthumously, in December 1956)
May 1956	Dr. Hajime Hosokawa notifies the Minamata public health office that four patients with neurological symptoms of unknown origin have been admitted to the Chisso hospital in Minamata (official identification of Minamata disease)
Aug. 1956	The Kumamoto University School of Medicine establishes a special research team to investigate Minamata disease
Jan. 1957	Kumamoto University researchers announce that the cause of Minamata disease is related to effluent con-

	taining heavy metals discharged by Chisso's Minamata plant
Aug. 1958	The Mutual Aid Association of the Families of Minamata Disease Patients is established
Sept. 1958	Chisso's Minamata plant switches its waste outlet from Hyakken Harbor to the mouth of the Minamata River, to the north
July 1959	Hosokawa begins experiments in which cats are made to ingest waste water from Chisso's Minamata plant
July 1959	Kumamoto University researchers announce that organic mercury (methyl mercury) is the causative agent of Minamata disease
Oct. 7, 1959	In Hosokawa's cat experiments, cat 400 exhibits symptoms of Minamata disease
Oct. 21, 1959	The Ministry of International Trade and Industry instructs Chisso to stop discharging waste water into the mouth of the Minamata River and to install purification equipment
Nov. 2, 1959	An investigative commission of Diet members visits Minamata; about 4,000 local fishers and sympathizers deliver a petition to the Diet members, march to the Chisso plant, and force their way in; they clash with police, and over 100 people are injured
Nov. 25, 1959	The Mutual Aid Association demands compensation of ¥3 million per patient from Chisso but is turned down
Nov. 28, 1959	Members of the Mutual Aid Association begin a sit-in in front of the main gate of Chisso's Minamata plant
Nov. 30, 1959	Chisso orders Hosokawa to discontinue his cat experiments
Dec. 19, 1959	Installation of equipment to purify waste water at Chisso's Minamata plant is completed, but waste water from the acetaldehyde production process does not pass through this equipment
Dec. 30, 1959	Members of the Mutual Aid Association sign a "condolence gift" agreement with Chisso
June 1960	Chisso resumes use of Hyakken Harbor as a waste outlet
July 1962	A labor dispute at Chisso's Minamata plant causes the labor union to split into the No. 1 Labor Union

	(opposed to management) and the No. 2 Labor Union (cooperative with management)
Feb. 1963	A Kumamoto University professor announces the discovery of organic mercury in sludge containing effluent from Chisso's Minamata plant
Jan. 1965	New Japan Nitrogen Co.'s name is changed to Chisso Corp.
June 1965	Niigata University School of Medicine researchers announce the discovery, along the Agano River, Niigata Prefecture, of patients with symptoms identical to those of Minamata disease
June 12, 1967	Families of patients of what is called Niigata Minamata disease file suit against the chemicals manufacturer Showa Denko with the Niigata District Court
Jan. 12, 1968	The Citizens' Council for Minamata Disease Countermeasures is established
Sept. 26, 1968	The central government officially declares mercury used in the production of acetaldehyde at Chisso's Minamata plant to be the cause of Minamata disease
Jan. 1969	*Kugai Jodo: Waga Minamata-byo* (Paradise of the Bitter Sea: My Minamata Disease), by Michiko Ishimure, is published
Apr. 15, 1969	The Association to Indict [Those Responsible for] Minamata Disease is established
Apr. 25, 1969	The Committee for Dealing with Minamata Disease Compensation is established
June 14, 1969	Twenty-nine families of Minamata-disease patients (112 people) file suit against Chisso with the Kumamoto District Court
Sept. 7, 1969	The Minamata Disease Study Group is established
Mar. 23, 1970	*Paradise of the Bitter Sea* is selected to receive the first Oya Prize for Nonfiction, but Michiko Ishimure declines the award
May 25, 1970	In Tokyo, the Compensation Committee presents its proposed settlement between Chisso and Minamata-disease patients; patients and members of the Association to Indict demonstrate in protest, and 13 people are arrested
June 28, 1970	The Tokyo chapter of the Association to Indict is established

July 4, 1970   Hosokawa, hospitalized for lung cancer, testifies from his hospital bed on his 1959 cat experiments

Oct. 13, 1970   Hosokawa dies

Nov. 28, 1970   Minamata-disease patients dressed as Buddhist pilgrims and 1,000 supporters holding one share of Chisso stock each attend the Chisso annual shareholders' meeting in Osaka and disrupt the proceedings

Sept. 29, 1971   The verdict in the Niigata trial is handed down; the plaintiffs are victorious

Oct. 6, 1971   Teruo Kawamoto is certified as a Minamata-disease patient

Nov. 1, 1971   Members of 18 families of Minamata-disease patients, including Kawamoto, begin a sit-in in front of the main gate of Chisso's Minamata plant to support their demand for ¥30 million in compensation for each patient

Dec. 7, 1971   Kawamoto and other representatives of Minamata-disease patients demanding direct negotiations with Chisso hand Chisso President Ken'ichi Shimada a list of demands at Chisso's Tokyo headquarters

Dec. 8, 1971   The patients demanding direct negotiations, together with members of the Association to Indict and other supporters, begin their struggle for direct negotiations at Chisso's Tokyo headquarters

Jan. 7, 1972   Workers at the Chisso plant in Goi, Chiba Prefecture, beat up Kawamoto and other members of the direct-negotiations group who are trying to meet with a union representative, as well as journalists covering the story

Oct. 15, 1972   Establishment of the Minamata Disease Center Soshisha is announced

Dec. 27, 1972   The Tokyo District Public Prosecutors Office indicts Kawamoto on the charge of infliction of bodily injury on Chisso employees

Mar. 20, 1973   The verdict in the Kumamoto trial is handed down; the plaintiffs are victorious

July 9, 1973   The Tokyo Chisso Negotiating Team (comprising the patients demanding direct negotiations and some of the victorious plaintiffs in the Kumamoto trial) and

Chisso sign a compensation agreement at the Environment Agency

Aug. 31, 1973   Michiko Ishimure receives the Magsaysay Prize

Apr. 7, 1974   The Minamata Disease Center Soshisha is completed

Jan. 13, 1975   The Tokyo District Court finds Kawamoto guilty of infliction of bodily injury; Kawamoto appeals the verdict; five members of families of Minamata-disease patients file charges of homicide and infliction of bodily injury against Chisso executives with the Tokyo District Public Prosecutors Office

Oct. 7, 1975   Two patients and two supporters are arrested, in Minamata and Kumamoto City, on suspicion of infliction of bodily injury and obstruction of the performance of official duties in connection with a protest on September 25 in Kumamoto City

Oct. 17, 1975   The four people arrested on October 7 are indicted on the charge of infliction of bodily injury

May 4, 1976   The Kumamoto District Prosecutors Office indicts Kiichi Yoshioka, former president of Chisso, and Eiichi Nishida, former manager of Chisso's Minamata plant, on the charge of infliction of death and bodily injury caused by negligence in the conduct of business

June 14, 1977   The Tokyo High Court overturns the Tokyo District Court's verdict against Kawamoto

June 15, 1977   The Tokyo High Public Prosecutors Office appeals the Tokyo High Court verdict, taking the case to the Supreme Court